'This is an innovative set of interventions to support practitioners helping young people to manage their aggression. It provides well-researched, detailed guides through a well-structured sequence of sessions. SHERBET fills an important gap in workshop provisions for youth workers.'

Professor David Canter, *Emeritus Professor at The University of Liverpool*

'The Mental Health Support Team in Nottingham City has piloted the SHERBET intervention since its creation. We have now run several groups and have seen significant positive impacts in terms of the benefits for children who find it hard to regulate their emotions. The intervention gives children an understanding of self, and allows them to explore strategies that work for them in a safe and supported environment.'

Dr Maddi Popoola, *Educational Psychologist and Mental Health Support Team Service Manager at Nottingham City Council*

Supporting Healthy Emotion Regulation and Behaviour Expression Treatment (SHERBET)

SHERBET is a unique tool designed to help practitioners support young people aged 11–17 who exhibit aggressive behaviours. Using CBT-based strategies, the programme aims to enhance their ability to recognise, regulate, and manage their emotions effectively.

Grounded in research and best practice, SHERBET draws on emotion regulation theories and motivational interviewing techniques. The structured group programme offers clear guidance in a supportive environment while remaining adaptable to individual needs. By addressing emotional overwhelm and unhealthy coping strategies early, the programme works to reduce future mental health and behavioural challenges.

Activities promote perspective taking, empathy development, and bias awareness, alongside strategies to strengthen communication skills. The comprehensive manual includes detailed instructions for staff training, programme evaluation, practical worksheets (also available as downloadable resources), and role-playing exercises for facilitating effective group sessions.

This resource is essential for all professionals working with children who experience difficulties with emotion regulation, including mental health practitioners, school counsellors, youth justice workers, social workers, special education teachers, and other professionals involved in child and adolescent well-being. Readers are expected to have a foundational understanding of child development, emotional and behavioural difficulties, and therapeutic interventions.

Sandra Jareño Ripoll is a forensic psychologist with experience working with both children and adults. Academically, her research focus has been youth knife offending and how to best tackle it. Through her research she has become passionate about promoting evidence-based practice, using research to inform the development and implementation of strategies and interventions. Dr Sandra Jareño Ripoll is also a practitioner psychologist, who has worked with children and adults, in the community and in custodial settings. Her experience has highlighted how beneficial early intervention, particularly regarding emotion recognition and regulation, can be for long-term outcomes.

Supporting Healthy Emotion Regulation and Behaviour Expression Treatment (SHERBET)

A Practical Guide to Reducing Aggressive Behaviour in Young People

Sandra Jareño Ripoll

Routledge
Taylor & Francis Group
LONDON AND NEW YORK

Designed cover image: Getty Images @Adrienne Bresnahan

First published 2026
by Routledge
4 Park Square, Milton Park, Abingdon, Oxon OX14 4RN

and by Routledge
605 Third Avenue, New York, NY 10158

Routledge is an imprint of the Taylor & Francis Group, an informa business

British Library Cataloguing-in-Publication Data
A catalogue record for this book is available from the British Library

ISBN: 9781041128144 (hbk)
ISBN: 9781041128120 (pbk)
ISBN: 9781003666738 (ebk)

DOI: 10.4324/9781003666738

Typeset in Times New Roman
by Newgen Publishing UK

Access the Support Material: https://resourcecentre.routledge.com/books/9781041128120

Dedicated to young people working toward brighter tomorrows, and to the professionals who stand with them every step of the way.

Contents

Preface

This intervention is designed to support practitioners working with young people to develop knowledge and skills related to managing emotions and behaviours. It is a structured, manualised intervention that can use to support young people in:

- recognising and regulating emotions
- problem solving and social skills
- mindfulness
- the influences and pressures that affect choices and behaviours
- how to manage these and make positive choices and decisions

Acknowledgements

This project would have not been possible without the unrelenting support and commitment from Nottingham's Mental Health Support Team. They believed in the value of SHERBET and helped it grow from an idea to a reality.

Thank you to Dr Sebrina Turner and Melanie Taylor, the sparks that lit the flame behind SHERBET and helped with the essential first steps to make it a reality. I send my thanks also to Georgina Blythe who accompanied me in those first steps.

My most sincere gratitude to Olivia Harvey, who always believed in the use, quality and future of SHERBET. Her creativity and contributions to the first draft were invaluable. Thank you for your excellent SHERBET delivery and training of staff which kept this intervention alive and in use beyond my stay in MHST. Specially, thank you for always making sure that I made space and time for myself too. I could not ask for a better collaborator and friend.

Thank you to Prof. Kevin Browne, who inspired me to be the best practitioner I can be. He held me up to high standards and ensured I held my own work to those same standards.

Thank you to all the young people and institutions who have embraced SHERBET so far, giving it their absolute best. Thank you for your trust and your feedback, which have helped this program grow into the best it can be.

Finally, thank you to my family, friends, and my wonderful husband, who kept me (mostly) sane throughout this process. SHERBET exists because they made sure I practiced what I preached.

My most sincere thank you to everyone who has been and will be involved with this project. I truly hope it brings value to the work of whose who deliver it and the lives of those who receive it.

1 Purpose of the Intervention

We all experience emotions – negative, positive, and everything in between. They are a part of our everyday lives. However, for some people, feeling these emotions can seem overwhelming, like an out-of-control roller coaster. Adolescents are particularly vulnerable to experiencing emotions in this way.[1] This feeling of being overwhelmed emotionally can lead to a deep need to do something that will stop the intensity. This can lead to unhealthy coping strategies and risky or challenging behaviours.[2,3] In the long-term, these experiences can increase the risk of developing mental health disorders,[4,5] displaying aggressive behaviour,[6] or being involved in the criminal justice system.[7]

The purpose of this intervention is to support young people with managing and regulating strong emotions when they feel overwhelming. Thompson (1994) defined emotion regulation as: 'the extrinsic and intrinsic processes responsible for monitoring, evaluating, and modifying emotional reactions, especially their intensive and temporal features, to accomplish one's goals' (p.28).[8] Essentially, emotion regulation describes a person's ability to effectively manage and respond to an emotional experience – some emotions may still feel like roller coasters, but they are no longer out of control.

Informed by reviews of the evidence base,[9,10] we have developed a group intervention which aims to support young people to develop emotion regulation skills. In addition to developing emotion regulation skills, this intervention aims to promote improved behavioural expression and communication. This may be achieved through exercises which promote perspective taking,[11] empathy,[11] bias awareness,[12] and communication.[13] This intervention also employs a Motivational Interviewing element, which promotes adherence[14] by ensuring that young people's goals are accounted for throughout the intervention. Overall, this intervention aims to provide young people with skills which allow them to regulate their emotions and behaviours, empowering them to take greater control over their lives and bring them closer to their goals.

This intervention is designed to support practitioners working with young people to develop knowledge and skills related to managing emotions and behaviours. It is a structured, manualised intervention that can use to support young people in:

- Recognising and regulating emotions
- Problem solving and social skills
- Mindfulness
- The influences and pressures that affect choices and behaviours
- How to manage these and make positive choices and decisions

DOI: 10.4324/9781003666738-1

References

1 Dahl, R.E. (2004). Adolescent brain development: A period of vulnerabilities and opportunities. *Annals of New York Academy of Sciences*, *1021*(1), 1–22.

2 Weiss, N.H., Tull, M.T., Davis, L.T., Searcy, J., Williams, I., & Gratz, K.L. (2015). A preliminary experimental investigation of emotion dysregulation and impulsivity in risky behaviours. *Behaviour Change*, *32*(2), 127–142.

3 Wallace, G.T., Henry, K.L., Barrett, K.C., & Conner, B.T. (2021). Personality and emotion dysregulation profiles predict differential engagement in a wide range of health-risk behaviors. *Journal of American College Health*, *71*(6), 1–13.

4 McLaughlin, K.A., Hatzenbuehler, M.L., Mennin, D.S., & Nolen-Hoeksema, S. (2011). Emotion dysregulation and adolescent psychopathology: A prospective study. *Behaviour Research and Therapy*, *49*(9), 544–554.

5 Aldao, A., Gee, D.G., De Los Reyes, A., & Seager, I. (2016). Emotion regulation as a transdiagnostic factor in the development of internalizing and externalizing psychopathology: Current and future directions. *Development and Psychopathology*, *28*(4pt1), 927–946.

6 Röll, J., Koglin, U., & Petermann, F. (2012). Emotion regulation and childhood aggression: Longitudinal associations. *Child Psychiatry & Human Development*, *43*, 909–923.

7 Kemp, K., Thamotharan, S., Poindexter, B., Barker, D., Tolou-Shams, M., & Houck, C.D. (2017). Emotion regulation as a predictor of juvenile arrest. *Criminal Justice and Behavior*, *44*(7), 912–926.

8 Thompson, R.A. (1994). Emotion regulation: A theme in search of definition. *Monographs of the Society for Research in Child Development*, *59*(2–3), 25–52.

9 Moltrecht, B., Deighton, J., Patalay, P., & Edbrooke-Childs, J. (2021). Effectiveness of current psychological interventions to improve emotion regulation in youth: A meta-analysis. *European Child & Adolescent Psychiatry*, *30*(6), 829–848.

10 Eadeh, H.M., Breaux, R., & Nikolas, MA. (2021). A meta-analytic review of emotion regulation focused psychosocial interventions for adolescents. *Clinical Child and Family Psychology Review*, *24*(4), 684–706.

11 Batanova, M.D., & Loukas, A. (2011). Social anxiety and aggression in early adolescents: Examining the moderating roles of empathic concern and perspective taking. *Journal of Youth and Adolescence*, *40*(11), 1534–1543.

12 Martinelli, A., Ackermann, K., Bernhard, A., Freitag, C.M., & Schwenck, C. (2018). Hostile attribution bias and aggression in children and adolescents: A systematic literature review on the influence of aggression subtype and gender. *Aggression and Violent Behavior*, *39*, 25–32.

13 Kislyakov, P., Shmeleva, E., Silaeva, O., Belyakova, N., & Kartashev, V. (2016). Indices of socio-emotional wellbeing of youth: Evaluation and directions of improvement. In *SHS Web of Conferences* (Vol. 28, p. 01056). EDP Sciences.

14 Lundahl, B.W., Kunz, C., Brownell, C., Tollefson, D., & Burke, B.L. (2010). A meta-analysis of motivational interviewing: Twenty-five years of empirical studies. *Research on Social Work Practice*, *20*(2), 137–160.

2 How to Use This Manual

The manual is designed to be used by facilitators working with young people aged 11–17 years. Those using the manual should have some experience of facilitating group and individual, therapeutically informed, work. It is beneficial for facilitators to have received some training on how to deliver this intervention (e.g. via joint delivery with an experienced facilitator), although appropriate planning and practice prior to session delivery may be sufficient.

This intervention includes a group information session, two individual 'goal setting' workshops (one before the group starts and one after), and 8 group sessions. There is some flexibility in the method of delivery:

- Individual 'goal setting' workshops are preferred. However, this may not always be possible. These sessions may be adapted into a group format to accommodate larger groups or young people who may struggle in a 1:1 setting.
- Group sessions may be adapted to a 1:1 format to support young people who have specific needs or may struggle in a group setting.
- Group sessions may be delivered once-weekly or twice-weekly. This depends on the needs and availability of the young people or host organisation*.

*For example, a once-a-week delivery allows the group to be completed within one school term. A twice-a-week delivery allows the group to be completed within one school half-term.

The relationship between the professional delivering treatment and the client receiving it (i.e. therapeutic alliance) can have an impact on treatment outcomes, such as dropout rates and symptom severity.[1, 2] It is therefore important for facilitators to build awareness of their own strengths and needs within a therapeutic space. For those who have never delivered this kind of work before it may be useful to do some background research on emotion regulation and challenging behaviours, as well as reflecting on their own values, beliefs, and motivations, and how these might impact their work with young people.

Another key challenge that facilitators will face is the discussion of sensitive topics as part of group delivery. These may include traumatic events, abuse and self-harm, amongst others. It is recommended that facilitators research the issues relevant to the young people in their target population, as they may be relevant experiences for attendees. Some relevant statistics include:

- 1 in 20 children in the UK have been sexually abused – this may be by adults or by peers.[3]
- Females ages 16–19 are 4 times more likely than the general population to be victims of rape, attempted rape, or sexual assault.[4]

DOI: 10.4324/9781003666738-2

- In the UK in 2018, there were 6,507 deaths by suicide (a rate of 11.2 deaths per 100,000 people).[5] It is estimated that 115 people are exposed to a single suicide, with one in five reporting that this experience had a devastating impact or caused a major life disruption.[6]
- The rate of deaths by suicide among under 25s increased by 23.7% in 2018 with Young men aged 15–24 being particularly at risk.[7]

Overall, facilitators are unlikely to know all that the young person in front of them has gone through. Nonetheless, facilitators may prepare themselves for this by being aware of the issues young people in their communities face. In fact, young people who have experienced trauma are more likely to develop emotion regulation difficulties,[8] increasing their likelihood of being referred to interventions like this one. It is therefore important to be sensitive about issues such as these and avoid victim-blaming language. Most importantly, facilitators must ensure they are familiar with the safeguarding procedures of their organisation, and follow these if any safeguarding concerns are raised.

Managing Challenges

It is important to ensure that facilitators are aware of and have considered how to manage challenges that may arise as a result of the content of this program.

Before beginning, facilitators should be familiar with organisational policy on how to handle significant disclosures that may come up during sessions (e.g. safeguarding, risk to self, risk to others, etc.). Attendees should be aware of the limits of confidentiality and the reasons for which facilitators may need to break confidentiality, for example:

- If information that suggests a client is at risk of harm (from self or others).
- If information suggests that another person is at risk of harm (from self, the client, or others).

It is advisable to *remind young people about the organisation's confidentiality policies before starting any work*. Facilitators should provide attendees with time and space to ask questions and discuss any issues they may have regarding processes. If a safeguarding concern needs to be raised, it can be beneficial to talk one-to-one with the young person regarding the concerns, so they understand why facilitators need to pass on the information. This approach can help preserve the trust of the client in facilitators, as they are less likely to feel 'betrayed' or that facilitators spoke 'behind their back'. This also allows for further support if the young person requires it.

Facilitators should ensure that young people are aware of the content of each session and that they can opt out if they become overwhelmed.

Facilitators should ensure that they *have adequate support and resources available for sensitive topics*. These may be flyers of local or national organisations that can support the young people if they have been affected by any of the topics discussed.

Facilitators should ensure that, if sensitive topics are addressed during the session, young people have the opportunity to engage in more light-hearted topics near the end of the session. This may support them to achieve a calmer emotional state before the session ends.

Taking a Collaborative Approach

It is important that the activities in the program are used as a way of generating dialogue with young people. The discussion that facilitators have with young people when taking part in the activities is where the real learning occurs; facilitators should ensure that they are as prepared for this as for the delivery of the activity.

It is also important to consider how to promote a collaborative approach and any barriers which may make this difficult. For example:

- Do you need to adapt any of the activities to make them more relevant to the experience of the young people you're working with?
- Do you need to adapt any resources or delivery styles to make the content easier to understand? Are you aware of and adapting to any learning or communication needs?
- Are the young people you're working with participating voluntarily? If not, how can you foster a respectful learning environment where they feel valued and treated as equal partners in the learning process?

Although the extent of its effectiveness has not been established, taking a collaborative approach has been linked to benefits for interventions with adolescents as they result in greater client satisfaction, engagement, attendance, and adherence.[9] A collaborative approach, where young people's opinions are valued and integrated into the program, may also improve their self-efficacy, autonomy, and self-esteem.

Collaborating with Organisations

Facilitators may be in collaboration with organisations when delivering the SHERBET program. Whether it be community teams, schools, youth justice services, or other organisations, it is likely that the delivery of SHERBET will occur within a host organisation. This host may provide participant referrals, facilities, and support staff, amongst other things.

Facilitators should endeavour to promote effective communication and collaboration with host organisations. This should promote the organisation's awareness and adherence to SHERBET principles. This, in turn, aims to improve the efficiency of SHERBET delivery, the support which the organisation can provide for attendees' needs, and attendees' ability to generalise skills beyond their sessions. Examples of this collaboration include:

- Awareness of the organisations safeguarding and confidentiality guidelines, as these may affect how facilitators respond to disclosures.
- Informing the organisation of dates and times of sessions, to ensure attendees are available and attending.
- Awareness or discussion of the organisation's exclusion policy (e.g. exclusions in schools, remand in youth justice) and how this may impact client attendance.
- Informing the organisation of helpful and unhelpful strategies identified in sessions, so they may avoid unhelpful responses and promote helpful strategies.

In order to support a collaborative approach with organisations, this manual provides the following resources for facilitators:

- A sample Service Level Agreement (SLA): This contains an information sheet on the purpose of the intervention and requirements for its delivery. This may be adapted depending on the needs of facilitators and the organisation.
- A sample closing report: This contains an outline of a feedback report for organisations covering outcomes, strengths and weaknesses of the delivery, and points for development in

future SHERBET deliveries (for both facilitators and the organisation). This sample report focuses on group delivery of SHERBET, although facilitators may use its structure to inform feedback for schools on individual sessions. This may be adapted depending on the needs of facilitators and the organisation. Feedback from facilitators so far suggests that the effort required for creating these reports may mean that they are not completed each time a group is run. However, the reports continue to be regarded as a valuable resource to support the organisation's commitment to SHERBET, meaning that such reports may be beneficial on a longer-term basis, such as quarterly.
- A 'Completer's Workbook': The workbook contains general sections on content covered, as well as tailored sections (e.g. 'emotion thermometer' worksheet) adapted to the unique needs of each young person. Organisations may use these tools to inform their support of attendees, promote effective communication with attendees, and encourage attendees to maintain the skills achieved (e.g. by reviewing content with them).

Session Delivery Considerations

Delivery Advice

SHERBET delivery can be adapted to the needs of clients and the host organisation. Although the program was conceived with group delivery in mind, session content was planned so it may be easily adapted to 1:1 delivery. Group sizes should be informed by the needs of clients (e.g. mental health, neurodiversity), facilitators (e.g. single facilitator or co-delivered) and the organisation (e.g. referral frequency, room size). Feedback from facilitators so far has suggested that groups may function best with a maximum of six clients per group.

As well as the size of the group, the clients within the group may impact delivery, as they may impact group dynamics. Group dynamics refers to the behavioural and psychological processes that take place within a social group.[10] This may include how people interact, communicate, influence each other, and work together.

Whenever possible, it is beneficial for facilitators to collaborate with the host organisation in the referral process. This may allow for referral to be sorted so individuals with wellknown pre-existing conflict may be allocated to different groups. This may improve engagement and reduce risk. However, it is not always possible to create this separation. In these cases it is essential that facilitators are informed of known group dynamics and associated risks. Facilitators may benefit from the following to manage group dynamics:

- Facilitators may use the Goal Setting Workshop to build rapport and engagement with each individual client. Within the workshop facilitators can also collaboratively establish clear goals and roles that will continue into the group setting. This clarity aligns expectations with clients, so they're more likely to sustain their adherence and commitment in the group setting.[11]
- Facilitators should use the Group Agreement (Session 1 Task 2) to establish clear group rules and, if appropriate, agree consequences to breaking the rules – this will guide behaviour and may help manage conflict before it arises.[12] Co-creating these ground rules increases client ownership of the rules and adherence to them. Facilitators may use their pre-existing knowledge of client needs and dynamics to suggest rules that they anticipate will be necessary.
- Facilitators' behaviour is key to role model and reinforce adherence to expectations, respect, and openness. Facilitators should foster inclusion and psychological safety by openly

encouraging diverse perspectives, normalising mistakes as part of learning, and intervening when these principles are challenged.[13]

- When conflict does take place facilitators should endeavour to address it constructively. In order to do this, facilitators should remain calm in their communication and refer back to the agreed group rules, clearly labelling the unacceptable behaviour.[14] Facilitators may wish to consider the function of the behaviour and support the child to use alternative prosocial behaviours to meet this function. Facilitators should consider the needs of each client and whether their behaviours can be addressed in the room or whether they need to be addressed in a 1:1 space (e.g. briefly step aside or outside).
- Facilitators should always consider practical factors that can increase safety and prevent conflict. For example, seating plans can create physical distance between people with pre-existing conflict. Additionally, facilitators will need to recognise if any items in the room need securing (e.g. it may not be appropriate to run a group in an art room where resources may be distracting, or sharps may be accessible).

Accessibility Advice

SHERBET aims to be an inclusive intervention, which can be delivered to a variety of populations. Accessibility has been at the core of SHERBET's framework and development. Resources and activities have been designed to be inclusive of communication needs, whilst still maintaining a comprehensive, structured and evidence-based approach.

SHERBET has adhered to Accessible Communication Guidelines,[15, 16] promoting accessibility to a greater number and variety of populations. Having an accessible standard format aims to reduce demand, and associated strain on facilitators, of developing special accessible versions. Any documents aimed at attendees have been adapted as follows:

- Written content, whenever possible, uses plain language (i.e. simple vocabulary and grammar).
- Headings and subheadings are used to provide structure and clarity.
- Key words are bolded in written content to enhance meaning.
- Written content is formatted using clear and easy to read fonts (e.g. avoiding cursive) and a minimum text size of 10 point.
- Visual cues are used throughout to enhance meaning.

Practitioners note: Although SHERBET's original documents aim to be widely accessible, some clients with visual impairments, learning disabilities, or literacy difficulties, may experience difficulties accessing some of the information in written text. It is expected that practitioners will have awareness of the communication needs of their client group and will adapt resources and delivery accordingly.

Task descriptions in the SHERBET manual highlight the evidence base and purpose of each task. Facilitators are therefore encouraged to adapt the format of the task if needed, whilst adhering to its evidence base and purpose. Some ways in which facilitators may adapt tasks include:

- Inserting additional visual cues – this may be done by editing worksheets or creating visual presentations (e.g. using a white board or PowerPoint) to accompany task explanations.
- Adapting the speed and complexity of spoken language.

- Promoting a welcoming environment where attendees feel valued and comfortable, so they may express when they need additional support or explanations.

Finally, if unsure, facilitators may seek support from supervisors, schools, and accessibility specialists to better understand and adapt to the needs of attendees.

References

1 Hawley, K.M., & Weisz, J.R. (2005). Youth versus parent working alliance in usual clinical care: Distinctive associations with retention, satisfaction, and treatment outcome. *Journal of Clinical Child and Adolescent Psychology, 34*, 117–128.

2 Ryan, R., Berry, K., & Hartley, S. (2023). Therapist factors and their impact on therapeutic alliance and outcomes in child and adolescent mental health–A systematic review. *Child and Adolescent Mental Health, 28*(2), 195–211.

3 NSPCC. (2019). *Child sexual abuse: statistics briefing.* NSPCC Available at: https://learning.nspcc.org.uk/research-resources/statistics-briefings/child-sexual-abuse/ [Accessed 5 November 2025].

4 Department of Justice, Office of Justice Programs, Bureau of Justice Statistics, Sex Offenses and Offenders (1997).

5 Office for National Statistics (2019). *Suicides in the UK: 2018 registrations.*

6 Cerel, J., Maple, M., van de Venne, J., Moore, M., Flaherty, C., & Brown, M. (2016). Exposure to suicide in the community: Prevalence and correlates in one US state. *Public Health Reports, 131*(1), 100–107.

7 Samaritans. (2019). *Suicide facts and figures.* [online] Available at: www.samaritans.org/about-samaritans/research-policy/suicide-facts-and-figures/ [Accessed 20 November 2019].

8 Villalta, L., Smith, P., Hickin, N., & Stringaris, A. (2018). Emotion regulation difficulties in traumatized youth: A meta-analysis and conceptual review. *European Child & Adolescent Psychiatry, 27*(4), 527–544.

9 Viksveen, P., Bjønness, S.E., Cardenas, N.E., Game, J.R., Berg, S.H., Salamonsen, A., Storm, M., & Aase, K. (2021). User involvement in adolescents' mental healthcare: A systematic review. *European Child & Adolescent Psychiatry, 31*, 1–24.

10 Forsyth, D. R. (2008). Group dynamics. In *Leadership: The key concepts*, edited by A. Marturano and J. Gosling (pp. 71–74). Routledge.

11 Tuckman, B.W., & Jensen, M.A.C. (2010). Stages of small-group development Revisited1. *Group Facilitation, 10*, 43.

12 Feldman, D.C. (1984). *The development and enforcement of group norms*. Academy of Management Review.

13 Edmondson, A. (1999). *Psychological safety and learning behavior in work teams*. Administrative Science Quarterly.

14 Johnson, D.W., & Johnson, R.T. (2000). *Conflict resolution and peer mediation programs in elementary and secondary schools: A review of the research.* Review of Educational Research.

15 GOV.UK. (2021). *Accessible communication formats.* [online] Available at: www.gov.uk/government/publications/inclusive-communication/accessible-communication-formats [Accessed 28 January 2022].

16 University Hospitals Sussex. (2022). Supporting staff and patients language and communication needs policy. University Hospitals Sussex. Available at: www.uhsussex.nhs.uk/wp-content/uploads/2022/10/Supporting-Staff-and-Patients-Language-and-Communication-Needs-Policy-1.pdf [Accessed 5 Dec 2025].

3 Post-Session Staff Debrief

Debriefing involves a structured process, which reviews the events and actions taken following an exercise. This can be valuable for facilitators, as it provides a forum to reflect on their experiences and improve their practice. The process of debriefing has been widely used in nursing and healthcare professions following simulations, to allow attendees to reflect on the events, solidify their learning, and plan for future situations. Although the literature on debriefing is limited and its methodology is varied, debriefing is overall seen as beneficial to the practice of professionals.[1, 2]

Following a session, facilitators should collaboratively debrief (a structured debrief sheet is provided in this manual's resources). This can improve the speed report writing, as a debrief allows for a space to discuss and summarize the content of the session and participation of attendees – these are both relevant when writing notes or reports. Staff debriefs are also likely to improve the detail and accuracy of such reports, as well as the overall awareness of what occurred in the session. This is because different staff members may have different conversations with attendees and may notice different comments and actions from them.

The debriefing session also allows for collaborative discussion of group dynamics, facilitator actions, and overall strengths and difficulties of the session. This allows for further adaptation, collaboration, and tailoring of sessions to improve future delivery and facilitator skills. In order for this to be effective, it is essential that debriefings are conducted with respect and an open mind. Feedback must be constructive and delivered in a tactful manner. Feedback must also be received in a tactful manner and seen as an opportunity to grow and improve one's practice.

Finally, the debrief session provides a valuable space to consider any risk and safeguarding issues. If any are present, plans on how to proceed should be made and recorded during the debrief meeting. A sample staff debrief structure may be found in the 'Worksheets and Resources' section.

References

1 Johnston, S., Coyer, F.M., & Nash, R. (2018). Kirkpatrick's evaluation of simulation and debriefing in health care education: A systematic review. *Journal of Nursing Education*, *57*(7), 393–398.

2 Dufrene, C., & Young, A. (2014). Successful debriefing—Best methods to achieve positive learning outcomes: A literature review. *Nurse Education Today*, *34*(3), 372–376.

DOI: 10.4324/9781003666738-3

4 Assessment and Evaluation

In order to review the effectiveness of the intervention, measures should be taken throughout. By measuring relevant factors we may track any changes or lack thereof, thus exploring the effectiveness of the intervention.

Measure Name	*What it measures*	*When to deliver it*
Behaviour and Feelings Survey (BFS)[1]	The BFS is well established as a measure for monitoring treatment response in children and adolescents. The measure counts with both youth report and caregiver report forms. It covers some relevant behavioural targets of the intervention such as emotional symptoms and conduct problems.	A youth and a caregiver measure should be completed prior to the beginning of the intervention (baseline) and after the final group session (end point). Measure outcomes may be discussed as part of the final Goals Workshop.
Difficulties in Emotion Regulation Scale – 14 item version (DERS-18)[2]	DERS-18 is a valid age-appropriate self-report measure designed to assess problems with emotion regulation.[3] It's a shorter version of the original 36-item DERS,[4] and it retains strong psychometric properties while being more time-efficient.	Should be completed by clients prior to the beginning of the intervention (baseline) and after the final group session (end point). Measure outcomes may be discussed as part of the final Goals Workshop.
Attendee Feedback and Reflection	During the final Goals Workshop young people are encouraged to reflect on their original challenges and goals, as well as their progress in overcoming them. Significant responses provide useful qualitative data on attendee perception of how effective the intervention was (e.g. their progress and how much SHERBET contributed to it)	During the final Goals Workshop.

DOI: 10.4324/9781003666738-4

Measure Name	*What it measures*	*When to deliver it*
Caregiver Feedback	This feedback questionnaire explores the caregiver's observations of change in attendee behaviour.	After the final Goals Workshop – within a week of SHERBET completion.
Host Organisation Feedback Sheet	This feedback questionnaire explores the host organisation's observations of change in attendee behaviour. It also covers feedback on the perceived quality and delivery of SHERBET (e.g. facilitator feedback, how easy it was for the organisation to accommodate the program), as these may be relevant factors impacting the effectiveness of the intervention.	After the final Goals Workshop – within a week of SHERBET completion.

It is also important to record any dropouts and the reasons for these. It may allow for identification of barriers to engagement in the intervention.

* *Please note that these tools may be used by practitioners as a guide to observe changes in emotion regulation following treatment but should not be considered a definite label or diagnosis. If these scores are shared with the young people or their family their limitations should be clearly highlighted.*

Outcome Measures – Facilitator Checklist

Facilitators may use the following checklist to ensure that they have collected the essential outcome measures as outlined above. It is acknowledged that not all facilitators will be able to engage caregivers or the Host Organisation in completing outcome measures. At the very least facilitators should endeavour to gather client measures to assess outcomes.

	Pre-SHERBET	*Post-SHERBET*
Client Measures	BFS – Youth DERS-18	BFS – Youth DERS-18
Caregiver Measures	BFS – Caregiver	BFS – Caregiver SHERBET Caregiver Feedback
Host Organisation Measures		SHERBET Host Organisation Feedback

References

1 Weisz, J.R., Vaughn-Coaxum, R.A., Evans, S.C., Thomassin, K., Hersh, J., Ng, M.Y., Lau, N., Lee, E.H., Raftery-Helmer, J.N., & Mair, P. (2020). *Behavior and Feelings Survey (BFS)* [Database record]. APA PsycTests.

2 Victor, S.E., & Klonsky, E.D. (2016). Validation of a brief version of the Difficulties in Emotion Regulation Scale (DERS-18) in five samples. *Journal of Psychopathology and Behavioral Assessment, 38*(4), 582–589. https://doi.org/10.1007/s10862-016-9547-9

3 Chen, Y.W.R., Janicaud, N., Littlefair, D., Graham, P., Soler, N., Wilkes-Gillan, S., ... & Cordier, R. (2024). A systematic review of self-regulation measures in children: Exploring characteristics and psychometric properties. *Plos One*, *19*(9), e0309895. doi: 10.1371/journal.pone.0309895

4 Gratz, K.L., & Roemer, L. (2004). Multidimensional assessment of emotion regulation and dysregulation: Development, factor structure, and initial validation of the difficulties in emotion regulation scale. *Journal of Psychopathology and Behavioral Assessment*, *26*(1), 41–54.

5 Duncan, B.L., Miller, S.D., Sparks, J.A., Claud, D.A., Reynolds, L.R., Brown, J., & Johnson, L.D. (2003). The Session Rating Scale: Preliminary psychometric properties of a "working" alliance measure. *Journal of Brief Therapy*, *3*(1), 3–12.

5 SHERBET's Research and Development Journey

Since its conception, SHERBET has aimed to be an evidence-informed and evidence-based information. The conceptual development of SHERBET has been evidence-informed, with each chapter's content being guided by research evidence and reference to this evidence being clearly linked and labelled. However, like any new intervention, SHERBET had to be applied for data on its impact to be collected and evaluated.

SHERBET collaborated with the Nottingham Mental Health Support Team (MHST) to deliver and evaluate the program. MHSTs are part of a national project that is NHS England funded and they offer a collaborative, system-wide approach to support the mental wellbeing of children in both Primary and Secondary schools and colleges. MHST staff were trained in the delivery of SHERBET and had access to the SHERBET manual.

Ethical Considerations

Consent was sought from the Head of Nottingham MHST to conduct an evaluation of the SHERBET intervention. The SHERBET evaluation considered data from children between the ages of 12–17, which requires parental consent for those children under the age of 18, as well as the thorough anonymization of data. MHST routinely uses a standard form to obtain 'Parental Consent to Share Information'. This form seeks consent for the collection and use of data for research purposes by external agencies and research groups. The existing consent-seeking process was therefore sufficient for the present programme evaluation.

To ensure participant privacy data for the evaluation was collected and collated by MHST staff, who anonymised the database prior to sharing it for the evaluation.

Pre- and post-intervention measures, as opposed to control group comparisons, were used for this study. MHSTs did not have an alternative intervention to tackle aggressive behaviours and prior to SHERBET they had been diverting young people with aggressive behaviours to other services. As a result, there was no 'treatment as usual' control group within MHST to allow for a fair comparison. Any control group would have implied a lack of access to treatment within MHST, which was considered unethical for this youth sample.

Data Sample

The sample evaluated consisted of young people referred by their school to the Nottingham City and County Mental Health Support Team (MHST) for support with anger and/or aggression, who were allocated to the SHERBET programme for intervention. Participants met the criteria for SHERBET if they were aged 11–17 and presented with anger management difficulties,

DOI: 10.4324/9781003666738-5

although these didn't need to be their primary problem (e.g. They may experience difficulties managing other emotions as well).

SHERBET was predominantly delivered in a group format (68%), with only a small number of young people being referred for 1:1 delivery (10%). Some young people received a blended approach (22%), where they may have started in a group format, but transitioned to 1:1 delivery depending on the young person or host organisation's needs (e.g. the school changed the schedule so group could not continue or young person missed a number of sessions due to illness). SHERBET was delivered in both mainstream schools (74%) and alternative schooling provisions (26%).

A total of 31 young people were referred to MHST meeting the criteria for SHERBET. Out of those referred, 18 (58%) completed the intervention. Reasons for deselection (13; 42% deselected) included participant illness (1, 8%), clashes in scheduling with school lessons (4; 31%), change in schools (2, 15%) and not believing that they'd benefit from the intervention (6, 46%).

Although the number of deselections is notable, this was significantly impacted by the context and timing. SHERBET was being developed and improved at the time of delivery, and it was noted that both the referral screening and the service level agreements could be strengthened. This is further explored in the section covering 'Feedback, Updates and Lessons Learned'.

Feedback and Lessons Learned

One of the areas explored in initial research was the quality of the delivery process of SHERBET, as measured by feedback from participants, referrer organisations, and facilitators. This process evaluation aimed to consider the factors impacting delivery of SHERBET, in order to best adapt and update the program following its initial development phase.

Facilitators provided feedback on the host organisation's adherence to the service level agreement (SLA), including an overall adherence score and written feedback. The SLA was introduced to host organisations to promote joint working and collaboration to increase the effectiveness of SHERBET (e.g. they agree to provide a safe uninterrupted space for sessions to take place, etc.). Participants contributed to process measures by providing written feedback on their experience of the SHERBET programme. Schools also provided written feedback of their experience of working with the SHERBET programme, as well as providing an overall satisfaction score.

To understand the feedback regarding the SHERBET program, we used thematic analysis, a method that helps organize and make sense of feedback in a structured way while still leaving space for flexibility. In practice, this meant carefully reading through responses and looking for patterns, repeated ideas, and meaningful differences.

The process began with one reviewer reading the feedback in detail and identifying key 'codes' – labels for important skills, reactions, or themes that appeared in participants' comments. A second reviewer, who had not been involved in running SHERBET, then reviewed the same data using these codes and their definitions. This step was important because it added another perspective and reduced the chance that the analysis was shaped too much by one person's assumptions. At this stage, both reviewers agreed on about three-quarters of the coding decisions (77%).

Next, the reviewers met to discuss where they had agreed and where their views differed. In this discussion, the second reviewer – who was unfamiliar with SHERBET – asked for clarification about which skills and activities were considered part of the program itself, and which were simply icebreakers or adaptations. This helped refine the coding system so it was clearer and more consistent. After updating the definitions and re-checking the responses, the reviewers reached full agreement (100%).

Finally, the individual codes were gathered into broader themes that reflected the main messages emerging from participants' feedback. Even codes that only appeared occasionally were kept in the analysis if they highlighted issues important for future delivery of SHERBET. Because the study involved a relatively small group, these less frequent but practically significant points were considered valuable to carry forward.

Attendee feedback. Out of the 18 young people who completed SHERBET, 17 provided feedback on their experience. The breakdown of the thematic analysis can be found in Table 5.1.

Attendee feedback primarily noted the helpfulness of SHERBET core content, mentioning specific gained tools and skills such as the emotion thermometer. Attendees in groups highlighted the impact of group interactions, both with peers and staff. Relationships with peers could have either a positive or negative impact. Good relationships with peers were noted as helpful whereas the presence of challenging peers or 'enemies' in the group made it difficult for attendees to engage. Although it was only briefly mentioned, the appropriateness of student referrals was also noted in facilitator feedback, whereby they reflected on the negative impact of placing young people with known problematic relationships in the same group.

Attendees' feedback of staff focused on their ability to manage behaviours in the group. This suggests it is important for facilitators to notice and respond to challenging behaviours and pre-existing negative relationships in the group. This allows facilitators to reduce the impact of challenges in group dynamics. Attendees also took notice of staff adaptations in the delivery of SHERBET. Feedback suggests that reasonable adaptations, aimed to target the needs and interests of participants, are valued and impactful.

Organisation feedback. Out of the 10 schools who hosted the SHERBET program, only five provided feedback on their experience of SHERBET. The breakdown of the thematic analysis can be found in Table 5.2. Organisation feedback highlighted that schools see SHERBET as both impactful and worth sustaining. Most organisations explicitly described SHERBET as beneficial for pupils. They noted that children enjoyed the sessions, gained coping strategies, and showed positive changes in behaviour. Several schools also expressed a desire to run the program again with new groups of pupils, indicating they saw lasting value in its continuation.

Organisations noted the importance of SHERBET staff's engagement with the host organisation's staff and students. All schools noted the impact of facilitators, whether it related to staff or students, noticing the importance of effective and collaborative facilitators. Organisations praised facilitators for the positive impact that positive relationships with staff and pupils had (e.g. engagement, problem-solving). It was suggested that increasing structured opportunities to share progress with school staff could further integrate SHERBET's benefits into the school environment.

Facilitator feedback. SHERBET facilitators provided feedback for all 10 schools who hosted the SHERBET program. The breakdown of the thematic analysis can be found in Table 5.3. Facilitator feedback highlighted the importance of the host organisation (e.g. school, AP, etc.) adhering to agreements and expectations both in and outside of sessions. For example, by providing a protected time for sessions (e.g. regular sessions, not prioritising other activities over sessions, not taking students out of session) and maintaining consistent communication with SHERBET staff (e.g. informing staff of cancelled sessions, providing a link member of staff for SHERBET communications). Protected time had a notable impact on the success of the program, contributing to inconsistent attendance and deselection when not provided and supporting adherence and engagement when provided.

Both in-session and out-of-session expectations are outlined in the SHERBET manual's service-level-agreement which facilitators are encouraged to review with the organisation hosting the SHERBET program prior to and during the delivery of SHERBET. Current feedback of the SHERBET delivery process highlights the need for facilitators to use the SLA to promote clarity of and adherence to expectations for organisations and staff involved in the delivery of SHERBET. The use of a clear SLA may also contribute to a continuing and strengthening the collaborative relationship with staff from the host organisations, highlighted in the feedback from host organisations.

Updates in Psychometric Measures

As outlined in the beginning of this chapter, SHERBET was always designed to be evidence-informed and evaluated. It was therefore recommended that all participants complete assessment and outcome measures, which would allow for evaluating the impact of the intervention. However, lessons learned have led to changes in the psychometric measures used to track outcomes.

Initially, the psychometric measures included the Emotion Regulation Questionnaire for Children and Adolescents (ERQ-CA)[1] and Strengths and Difficulties Questionnaire (SDQ).[2]

Systematic reviews of interventions for emotion regulation had highlighted that most emotion regulation interventions failed to include an appropriate emotion regulation assessment in their evaluations.[3, 4] The inclusion of an emotion regulation measure was therefore considered essential to assess whether SHERBET was properly addressing emotion regulation skills, assessing its face validity.

The ERQ-CA was chosen because it is a valid age-appropriate measure for investigating the use of emotional suppression and cognitive reappraisal in children and adolescents. It shows strong psychometric properties including test-retest reliability.[1, 5] This implied that significant changes to scores may be an accurate reflection of the impact of interventions. Instructions in the ERQ-CA ask participants to focus on how they currently manage their emotions when answering the questionnaire. This allows for a brief snapshot of their skills, which can then be compared to their scores following treatment.

However, consistent feedback from attendees and facilitators suggested that, despite the ERQ-CA being designed for young people between the ages of 10–18, attendees often failed to understand the complexly worded items. Participants regularly reported difficulty comprehending and responding to the ERQ-CA. This likely impact the validity of outcomes, as young people were not able to provide accurate responses. It was therefore decided that SHERBET would benefit from a different, more accessible, measure assessing for emotion regulation. The replacement measure was the 18-item version of the Difficulties in Emotion Regulation Scale 18 (DERS-18).[6] A systematic review of emotion regulation measures in children[7] identified the DERS and its brief version as being the most extensively researched self-report measure exploring emotion regulation skills in children and adolescents aged 11–17. It was noted by facilitators that this measure also showcased better face validity. Questions were more accessible and more easily understood, therefore being more likely to result in accurate responses from participants.

The SDQ was initially chosen as an outcome measure because it is a brief, reliable and valid measure which explores the adjustment and psychopathology of children and adolescents, covering both internalising and externalising conducts.[2] The SDQ shows good psychometric properties (e.g. internal consistency, test-retest, linked to mental health diagnoses[2]).

This measure aimed to assess the practical impact of SHERBET on the child's ability to manage their anger and other emotions. Scores were gathered at the start and end of intervention to allow for comparison assessments. However, this tool was not sensitive enough to measure change across an 8–10 week period. The SDQ instructs participants to consider the presence of questionnaire items over the last 6 months. The length of time period covered makes it unlikely that significant changes will be reflected following the 8–10 weeks of intervention.

The selected replacement for the SDQ was the Behaviour and Feelings Scale (BFS), which is established as a measure for monitoring treatment response in children and adolescents.[8] Positively, the BFS also shows strong psychometric properties (e.g. robust factor structure, internal consistency, test-retest reliability, convergent and discriminant validity[7]). The BFS, like the SDQ, measures internalising and externalising behaviours in young people. Also, like the SDQ, the measure counts with both youth report and caregiver report forms. Notably, the main improvement of the BFS is that it asks respondents to focus on the presence of problems in the last week – this shorter time period would increase sensitivity and may more accurately reflect changes following intervention.

Impact and Outcomes

The impact of SHERBET was investigated, exploring whether SHERBET is effective in supporting positive change in young people with emotion regulation difficulties. Unfortunately, as outlined, the initial psychometrics were not considered appropriate for evaluating the intervention, and so they were not included in this first evaluation. The impact of SHERBET was measured using referrer ratings (i.e. intensity of problem behaviour before and after SHERBET) and qualitative feedback from referrers and participants.

SHERBET participants were included in the evaluation if they had completed SHERBET and had complete outcome measures (i.e. referrer ratings and feedback from referrers and participants). A total of 17 young people met the criteria and were considered in this evaluation. Participants were aged between 12 and 15 years old (Mean age: 12.88). The sample included 6 (35%) female and 11 (65%) male participants. 3 participants (18%) had diagnosed special educational needs, such as Autism Spectrum Disorder (ASD) and Attention Deficit Hyperactivity Disorder (ADHD).

A paired samples sign test was conducted to determine the effect of the SHERBET programme on referrer's ratings of the intensity of problem behaviours. The paired samples sign test is a non-parametric alternative to a paired-samples t-test. This allows for calculations to compare smaller samples such as the ones present in the SHERBET evaluation. The results showed significant differences in the intensity of problem behaviours as rated by referrers (i.e. school staff) before and after SHERBET ($z=4.12311$, $p<0.01$).

It was also recorded whether participants required a referral for further support at the end of treatment. Out of 17 respondents, 15 (88%) did not need further support from services after completion of SHERBET. Two participants requested further support regarding anxiety.

We also explored qualitative feedback provided by young people and host organisations, asking them to reflect on changes in the young person's behaviour following the completion of SHERBET. A thematic analysis was conducted on this feedback and a number of themes were identified.

The setting and reviewing of goals are key elements of SHERBET, so it is not surprising that all 17 young people referred to their goals when considering their progress. The primary goal focus was the management of challenging emotions, with specific mentions of anger (n= 7, 41%) and distraction (n=4, 24%). Participants also described behavioural elements to their goal, discussing changes in challenging behaviours (n=7, 41%) such as becoming physically aggressive and walking out of class. A number of participants also mentioned consequences (n= 4, 24%), such as detentions or exclusions, and wanting to reduce how often they got 'in trouble'. This suggests that these are effective measures by which they track their progress.

All 17 young people reported improvement in their goals (100%), with most recognising that they still had room for improvement (n=14, 82%). Considering that only a small minority of attendees required further involvement from mental health services, these results suggest that participants were realistic that their behaviour, despite improvement, was not 'perfect' but it was manageable.

Feedback from host organisations (Table 5.4) also noted significant improvements in young people who participated in SHERBET. This primarily included a reduction in problem behaviours, such as aggression, violence, and 'emotional outbursts' (n=16, 94%). Improvements were also noticed in participants wellbeing (n=8, 47%), with feedback noting signs of improved wellbeing such as better emotion recognition, reductions in low mood, and a more relaxed presentation. Host organisations specifically noted improvements in young people's relationship and communication with staff (n=10, 59%) and their use of strategies learned in SHERBET (n= 6, 35%). Nonetheless, some outstanding behavioural issues were identified, suggesting some ongoing difficulties with problem behaviours despite improvements (n=6, 35%).

Overall, host organisations reported a significant decrease in the intensity of problem behaviours following participation in the SHERBET program, and qualitative feedback from both attendees and schools noted improvements in internal experiences (e.g. increased emotion control, improved wellbeing) and externalising behaviours (e.g. reports of disruptive behaviour). Both attendees and schools also highlighted the use of SHERBET strategies as contributing to positive changes.

Conclusions and Next Steps

The initial evaluation of SHERBET provides promising evidence that it can support young people in developing emotion regulation skills and reducing problem behaviours. Although the evaluation was exploratory in scope, findings consistently indicated that SHERBET is both acceptable to participants and feasible for delivery within structured environments, such as schools and APs. Importantly, both young people and host organisations highlighted the relevance of SHERBET's tools, the value of supportive group processes, and the positive impact on behaviour and wellbeing.

The evaluation also revealed several challenges that offer direction for improvement – informing updates in the SHERBET manual and providing guidance to practitioners. High rates of deselection and attendance difficulties were influenced by factors such as scheduling clashes, referral processes, and group dynamics. Strengthening referral screening and clarifying expectations with host organisations through service-level agreements may reduce attrition and improve engagement. Feedback also underscored the importance of facilitators being responsive to group dynamics and of ensuring that schools provide protected time and space for consistent delivery.

Methodologically, the evaluation highlighted the need for more accessible and sensitive outcome measures. The adoption of the DERS-18 and the Behaviour and Feelings Scale (BFS) reflects an important step towards more valid and reliable assessments of SHERBET's impact on young people's emotion regulation and behavioural outcomes. Future evaluations will benefit from the improved psychometric alignment between intervention aims and outcome measures.

Taken together, the findings suggest that SHERBET is a promising intervention with potential to address a critical service gap in the support of young people experiencing difficulties managing anger and aggression. However, further development and rigorous evaluation are required.

Regarding delivery, adaptations have already been made to the SHERBET manual to reflect the knowledge gained by this research, such as updating the recommended psychometric tools and increasing guidance on managing group dynamics. It is recommended that future practitioners using SHERBET remain aware of the factors impacting service delivery, endeavouring to adapt their practice to ensure that these factors are sufficiently addressed. Ongoing gathering of data will also be beneficial for future research on service delivery, ensuring that SHERBET remains responsive to the needs of diverse learners and settings.

Regarding the evaluation of SHERBET's impact and outcomes, it will be essential for further research to be carried out, incorporating the newly recommended psychometric measures. In most cases this will focus on comparing participant scores before and after completion of SHERBET. However, where ethical and appropriate, control groups may be used to strengthen causal inferences about SHERBET's effectiveness. The present manual and overall SHERBET project aims to support research efforts by collating anonymised data gathered by practitioners. The present manual includes resources (e.g. psychometric measures, blank data table) to support the gathering of anonymised outcome data which SHERBET authors may collate to continue research efforts.

In conclusion, SHERBET demonstrates encouraging early outcomes as an evidence-informed intervention targeting anger and emotion regulation difficulties in young people. With continued refinement, systematic evaluation, and strengthened implementation processes, SHERBET has the potential to become an established, evidence-based programme that supports both the emotional wellbeing and behavioural adjustment of adolescents across education settings.

Table 5.1 Breakdown of themes and codes identified from attendee feedback on SHERBET delivery. The table includes the definitions of themes and codes, the frequency of mentions for each theme and code, and sample quotes to illustrate the content of the themes and codes.

Theme (number of mentions/ total responses) and Definition	*Code (number of mentions/total responses) and Definition*	*Quotes*
SHERBET Core Content (14/18): Attendee perceptions of the core content of SHERBET (i.e. elements included in the SHERBET manual as content/strategies to cover in sessions). This theme covers strengths and areas of development in the SHERBET core content.	**Tools/Skills (14/18):** Attendee mentions tools/skills taught in the SHERBET program – may be positive or negative feedback.	'I liked the emotion thermometer. It was helpful because it helped me reflect on how I was feeling and give me some helpful ideas to feel better' 'Traffic lights helped me to easily communicate I needed I break. It was a quick way to show what I needed'. 'Activities(strategies)—glad it was a range rather than just deep breaths, made them fun. Like different puzzles and ways of learning'.

(*Continued*)

Table 5.1 (Continued)

Theme (number of mentions/ total responses) and Definition	*Code (number of mentions/total responses) and Definition*	*Quotes*
	Icebreakers/engagement activities (4/18): Attendee mentions activities included in the SHERBET program/manual which are not specifically emotion regulation/skill based—may be positive or negative feedback.	'I liked the skittle game'. *(Describes skittles icebreaker activity)*
SHERBET Delivery Style (7/18): Attendee perceptions of the delivery format of SHERBET. The SHERBET manual allows for and encourages the adaptation of SHERBET delivery to meet the needs of attendees (e.g. group vs 1:1 format, use of breaks, accessibility adaptations). This theme covers strengths and areas of development in the SHERBET delivery format and adaptations.	**Delivery Format (3/18):** Attendee comments regarding the delivery format and how this impacted their experience (e.g. size of group, group vs 1:1) – may be positive or negative feedback.	'Good being 1-1' 'I liked that there was not lots of people-the small numbers gave me chance to get close to them and talk to them, rather than thinking "can I say this in front of 30 people?" '
	Adaptations made (6/18): Attendee comments on adaptations made to the delivery of SHERBET to meet the group's needs (e.g. use of breaks, re-engagement activities, accessibility) – may be positive or negative feedback.	'Having the option to do worksheets on laptop as struggle with writing. Liked when break was cut shorter so we could do more work'. 'I liked that when we got a question right we got a gummy – I liked being competitive and thinking quickly'. 'I liked that we changed to have a break at the end to play football' 'Would change sessions to being in the morning, I feel more awake'
Group interactions (8/18): Attendee descriptions of group interactions in sessions, including relationships with peers and staff.	**Behaviour management (6/18):** Attendee comments on staff's ability or methods for managing behaviour of attendees in session – may be positive or negative feedback.	'School staff told *(other student)* off if he was mean'. 'Think SHERBET facilitator could have told *(other student)* off more' The facilitators were 'nice and kind'
	Peer relationships (8/18): Attendee comments on behaviours of and relationships with other group attendees.	'The small numbers gave me chance to get close to them and talk to them' 'I have liked having people to talk to about how I am feeling' 'What was something you did not like about SHERBET: People there with me – don't get on with them outside of class'. 'Made new friends (…) Was weird as enemies in the group. Don't think I'll stay friends with them'.

Table 5.2 Breakdown of themes and codes identified from organisation feedback on SHERBET delivery. The table includes the definitions of themes and codes, the frequency of mentions for each theme and code, and sample quotes to illustrate the content of the themes and codes.

Theme (number of mentions/ total responses) and Definition	*Code (number of mentions/total responses) and Definition*	*Quotes*
SHERBET Effectiveness (3/5): Perceptions of the host organisation which show a judgement on the effectiveness of the SHERBET program.	**Attendee impact (3/5):** Description of the extent of impact SHERBET has had on attendees and their behaviours.	'Our pupils have enjoyed and gained so much from the sessions' 'This group has been a massive success for the School. Our children have really benefited from the sessions and it really shows in their data'. 'Pupils seemed to really enjoy it. Gave them coping strategies to move forward with'.
	Wanting to run the group again (3/5): The host organisation expressing a desire to run the group again with another cohort of attendees.	'We have decided to continue holding the SHERBET sessions in our school for the foreseeable future' 'Am hopeful we can offer this to more of our pupils'
SHERBET Delivery 5/5): Host organisation's feedback on the way that students and staff were engaged in the delivery of SHERBET.	**Facilitator impacts on students (3/5):** Host organisation's feedback on SHERBET facilitators' strengths and areas of improvement in relation to work with students.	'The facilitators were absolutely amazing and ran the group perfectly. They both built up great relationships with all of the children in the group'. (*would like*) 'More 1-1 sessions at the start to build relationships before going into group sessions'. 'The practitioners were great with the students and did lots of varied activities to engage them'.
	Staff engagement (3/5): Host organisation's feedback on SHERBET facilitators' strengths and areas of improvement in relation to work with staff.	'Might be good to meet the pupils tutors at some point – start, mid way, end – maybe sharing' 'Regular feedback with the Achievement Leader (Head of Year about behaviour and challenges'. 'I feel the wider impact is that the facilitator worked closely with myself meaning additional SEND support was set up around both pupils which has hopefully helped improve the school environment for the two pupils involved'

Table 5.3 *Breakdown of themes and codes identified from facilitator feedback on SHERBET delivery. The table includes the definitions of themes and codes, the frequency of mentions for each theme and code, and sample quotes to illustrate the content of the themes and codes.*

Theme (number of mentions/ total responses) and Definition	*Code (number of mentions/ total responses) and Definition*	*Quotes*
Adherence to in-session expectations (10/10): Facilitator feedback on the extent of the host organisation's adherence to agreements and expectations that promote attendees' physical and psychological safety in sessions.	**Protected time (4/10):** Descriptions of the organisation's adherence to protecting time for sessions to take place at consistent, agreed times.	'protected session times'. 'When child was in school supported to attend sessions' 'Interrupted sessions to take students out. Poor timetabling prioritised activities other than SHERBET and led to group being discontinued'. 'Students being excluded/suspended, even after multiple conversations, requests and meetings where agreed no suspensions on day of SHERBET'.
	Protected Space (3/10): Descriptions of the organisation's adherence to protecting a space for sessions to take place at a consistent, safe, agreed space.	'Room was appropriate for sessions and was able to lock the room during break'. 'at points staff and pupils would walk in to talk to other staff/pupils which could cause a certain level of distraction – after discussing this with staff member this happened less'
	Staff involvement in sessions (4/10): Organisation's ability to adhere to agreements regarding staff involvement in sessions, such as whether staff would or wouldn't be present in the room during sessions and the extent of their contributions in sessions.	'Sometimes teachers would swap part way through a session. Young people responded differently to different teachers so were some problems managing behaviour in certain sessions'. 'Interrupted sessions to take students out'.
	Appropriateness of student referrals (2/10): Organisation's ability to adhere to agreements regarding students included in the group e.g. appropriateness of referral behaviours and consideration of group dynamics.	'problems with group dynamics, however, upon discussing this with school staff understand that this can be a difficult request in an SEMH school'.

Table 5.3 (Continued)

Theme (number of mentions/ total responses) and Definition	*Code (number of mentions/ total responses) and Definition*	*Quotes*
Adherence to out-of-session expectations (5/10): Organisation's adherence to agreements for out-of-session staff behaviours, such as maintenance of skills in students and collaboration with SHERBET staff.	**Consistent communication (7/10):** Organisation's ability to maintain appropriate communication as agreed with SHERBET staff.	'Was one allocated staff member for communications – staff member would make time to talk through any concerns or queries and assisted with any printing or other requests'. 'not making practitioner aware when young person was not in'. 'Link worker went off sick and no one else was able to replace/support with sessions or maintenance outside of sessions'
	Promoting skill use (4/10): School's ability to support the generalisation of skills learnt in SHERBET outside of sessions e.g. supporting students to use skills, promoting engagement in skills and sessions.	'Promoted positive view of SHERBET'. 'Initially it was agreed that instead of someone being in the session facilitator would send a follow up email after for students' key workers to follow up with students – this was not happening. Tweaked agreement so that key worker would come in for last 10 minutes for students to give recap which was more effective for students' retention and maintenance'. 'The same staff attended the group each week (…) meaning support was available out of sessions'.

Table 5.4 Breakdown of themes and codes identified from attendee feedback on SHERBET outcomes. The table includes the definitions of themes and codes, the frequency of mentions for each theme and code, and sample quotes to illustrate the content of the themes and codes.

Theme (number of mentions/ total responses) and Definition	*Code (number of mentions/ total responses) and Definition*	*Quotes*
Description of participant goals (17/17): Participants refer to specific goals for what they wish to achieve in treatment.	**Goal targets for anger (7/17):** Participant goals make reference to the management of anger.	'Learn to be more careful/control anger' 'Continuing to controlling anger and improving. When I get angry don't take it out on other people'
	Goal targets for distraction (4/17): Participant goals make reference to the management of distraction.	'To get less distracted, less zoning out, less moving/restless' 'Stop getting in to fights, better behaviour and concentrate more at school. Initially 5/10 end 7/10'.

(*Continued*)

Table 5.4 (Continued)

Theme (number of mentions/ total responses) and Definition	*Code (number of mentions/ total responses) and Definition*	*Quotes*
	Goal targets for challenging behaviours (7/17): Participant goals make reference to the management of challenging behaviours, such as becoming physically aggressive and walking out of class.	'Stop getting in to fights, better behaviour and concentrate more at school'. 'Don't want to be hitting stuff'
	Goal targets for consequences (4/ 17): Participant goals make reference to consequences, such as detentions or exclusions.	'Wanting to get in less troubles'. 'Got excluded 14 times last year. Only once this year (6 months into school term)'
Description of participant improvement (17/17): Host organisation feedback which highlights specific factors which have contributed to improvements in problem behaviours and wellbeing following SHERBET completion.	**Participants describing improvement in their goals (17/17):** Participants note positive improvement relating to their goals following completion of SHERBET.	'Feel like my anger has got better. Would shout at teachers and get detentions. I think this is because of SHERBET. We have helped me to think about how I speak to people and what I want to achieve from conversations with them – shouting is not always the best, particularly with staff'. 'I have had no detentions. I have not got as angry. 'Learn to be more careful/control anger – At start was a 5 end a 10'.
	Room for Improvement (14/17): Participants note room for improvement or outstanding difficulties following completion of SHERBET.	'In SHERBET I have improved my concentration. I find this hard in other lessons'. 'I am getting less detentions, but I still have more warnings. This is for stupid things like talking, rocking on my chair. But anger is better'. 'Continuing to controlling anger and improving. Start 5 now 8'. 'goal: walking out of lesson less (started 5/10, mid way 9/10, now 7/10)'

Table 5.5 Breakdown of themes and codes identified from host organisation feedback on SHERBET outcomes. The table includes the definitions of themes and codes, the frequency of mentions for each theme and code, and sample quotes to illustrate the content of the themes and codes.

Theme (number of mentions/ total responses) and Definition	*Code (number of mentions/ total responses) and Definition*	*Quotes*
Participant progress (17/ 17): Perceptions of the host organisation regarding the progress/changes made by participants following SHERBET completion.	**Reduction in problem behaviours (16/ 17):** The host organisation describing improvements in participants' behavioural difficulties.	'Relationships with other students have improved – not as many fall outs in playground'. 'has had no recorded incidents since leaving the group'. 'Overall behaviour has improved and scholar has been calmer around his peers. Reduction in number and frequency of behavioural incidents around the academy'.
	Improvements in participant wellbeing (8/17): The host organisation describing improvements in participants' wellbeing.	'He's having more fun – not so serious. Interacting with others in a more relaxed way'. 'The change in C's demeanour has been profound. He is much brighter in himself, happier and positive about all aspects of school'. 'Has made improvements of understanding her emotions and how she feels'.
	Outstanding concerns (6/17): The host organisation identifying participants having outstanding behavioural issues.	'has still struggled with cooperating with staff if he does not agree with a decision and he still displays aggressive behaviour. However, he has shown that he can use some strategies to avoid going into crisis'. 'Although he displayed some of the aggressive behaviours, he showed a calmer approach to conversations with staff and used strategies' 'needs to improve on how to regulate her emotions and being more resilient'
Factors contributing to improvement (10/17): Host organisation feedback which highlights specific factors which have contributed to improvements in problem behaviours and wellbeing following SHERBET completion.	**Participants' relationship and communication with staff (10/17):** Host organisation describes improvements in the young person's relationship with staff, such as improved trust or communication.	'more often than not, he cooperates with staff on a one-to-one basis. This is a marked improvement compared to summer term'. 'Before, if he was upset about something he could become angry and was very difficult to approach whereas now, he is very reasonable, understanding, considerate and mature'.
	Staff engagement (6/ 17): Host organisation describes the use of SHERBET strategies which have been helpful to staff and/or participants.	'Willing to take on advice and techniques given during sherbet programme, therefore, will help him regulate behaviour and emotions'. 'He is also better at removing himself from a situation before he acts in a way he may regret, showing improved self regulation and preventative strategies'.

References

1 Gullone, E., & Taffe, J. (2012). The emotion regulation questionnaire for children and adolescents (ERQ–CA): A psychometric evaluation. *Psychological Assessment*, *24*(2), 409. doi: 10.1037/a0025777

2 Goodman, R. (2001). Psychometric properties of the strengths and difficulties questionnaire. *Journal of the American Academy of Child & Adolescent Psychiatry*, *40*(11), 1337–1345. https://doi.org/10.1097/00004583-200111000-00015

3 Moltrecht, B., Deighton, J., Patalay, P. et al. (2021). Effectiveness of current psychological interventions to improve emotion regulation in youth: A meta-analysis. *European Child & Adolescent Psychiatry*, *30*, 829–848. https://doi.org/10.1007/s00787-020-01498-4

4 Eadeh, H.M., Breaux, R., & Nikolas, M.A. (2021). A meta-analytic review of emotion regulation focused psychosocial interventions for adolescents. *Clinical Child and Family Psychology Review*, *24*, 684–706. https://doi.org/10.1007/s10567-021-00362-4

5 Ioannidis, C.A., & Siegling, A.B. (2015). Criterion and incremental validity of the emotion regulation questionnaire. *Frontiers in Psychology*, *6*, 247. doi: 10.3389/fpsyg.2015.00247

6 Victor, S.E., & Klonsky, E.D. (2016). Validation of a brief version of the Difficulties in Emotion Regulation Scale (DERS-18) in five samples. *Journal of Psychopathology and Behavioral Assessessment*, *38*, 582–589. https://doi.org/10.1007/s10862-016-9547-9

7 Chen, Y.W.R., Janicaud, N., Littlefair, D., Graham, P., Soler, N., Wilkes-Gillan, S., ... & Cordier, R. (2024). A systematic review of self-regulation measures in children: Exploring characteristics and psychometric properties. *Plos One*, *19*(9), e0309895. doi: 10.1371/journal.pone.0309895

8 Weisz, J.R., Vaughn-Coaxum, R.A., Evans, S.C., Thomassin, K., Hersh, J., Ng, M. Y., … Mair, P. (2019). Efficient monitoring of treatment response during Youth Psychotherapy: The behavior and feelings survey. *Journal of Clinical Child & Adolescent Psychology*, *49*(6), 737–751. https://doi.org/10.1080/15374416.2018.1547973

6 Breaking the Ice

Icebreakers can be an effective way to build rapport between young people and facilitators. This can help the young people to feel more comfortable participating in the sessions and improves engagement.[1] Icebreakers also allow the facilitator to learn more about the young people they are working with through informal means.[2] Facilitators should actively take part in the icebreakers – this allows young people to build trust, familiarity, and good working relationships with facilitators.[3] It's important to let young people know they have a choice as to how much they participate in these activities.

Timings have been estimated on a group of 6–8 young people. Facilitators can adapt times according to the number and needs of the group.

Introductions and 'Getting to Know You'

Name, Pronoun, and Icebreaker Question

Duration: 10–15 Minutes

Resources: N/A

This is a quick introduction activity that promotes discussion of the young person's interests.

The facilitator should explain that they will be asking for names, pronouns, and using an icebreaker question. Some exploratory questions may include:

- What is your favourite ...
  - Film/TV programme
  - Food
  - Drink
  - Place to be
  - Country
  - Animal
- If you were a ... what ... would you be? And why?
  - Vegetable
  - Animal
  - Plant
  - Chocolate
  - Game console

DOI: 10.4324/9781003666738-6

It is recommended to use one question per session.

The facilitator should remind young people they do not have to explain 'why' if they choose not to. Moreover, the facilitator should allow for conversation between young people as this can be a good way for them to identify shared interests. Young people can also be encouraged to think of their own questions for the icebreaker.

Check-Ins (Can Also be Done with Introductions)

What... Are You Today?

Duration: 10 Minutes

Resources: Check-in images

This can be a fun way to check how young people are feeling.

The facilitator should use appendix 1 or make their own. They can then ask the young person to choose the number or point at the picture that best represents how they are feeling. Young people should be encouraged to discuss why they chose the picture but should not be pressured to do so. Some young people struggle to name emotions. By giving them the opportunity to choose a picture it reduces pressure on the person to name the emotions and helps build their confidence for future sessions.

The handout may be adapted to feature different images such as:

- Emojis
- Dogs
- Cats
- Racoons
- Memes
- Pictures of well-known characters such as Harry Potter, Shrek, SpongeBob, etc.

The facilitator may also ask the young people if there are any themes they would like to find for future sessions.

Poop Sandwich

Duration: 15 Minutes

Resources: N/A

The facilitator should explain to young people that they will be making a 'poop sandwich'. This activity involves sharing one good thing that happened in the last week or so, one bad thing, then another good thing (the 2 positives are the bread and the negative is the filling of the sandwich).

This check-in allows young people the space to share if they have had any negative experiences the last week whilst highlighting the positive.

Team Building

The following activities allow young people to get to know more about each other and the facilitators.

2 Truths 1 Lie

Duration: 20 Minutes

Resources: Pen, Paper

The facilitator should ask the young people to think of 2 truths and 1 lie, they should be told to keep these private but informed that they will be asked to share these with the rest of the group shortly. It can be helpful to give young people a few minutes to plan their statements as well as paper and pen so they may remember what they have chosen.

Once the facilitator has given sufficient time for people to think, they should explain they will be asking them to share their truths and a lie with the group – the aim is for the other members of the group to guess which story is a lie, and for the person sharing to disguise this as best as possible.

For example, someone might say:

- I love Video games
- I love Football
- I love Sushi

Two of these would be the truthful, and the young people have to guess which one is a lie.

Would You Rather?

Duration: 10–15 Minutes

Resources: N/A

This activity can be delivered through different methods; a) standing debate or b) stand and sit.

a) Standing debate: First ensuring that there is adequate space, the facilitator should ask the young people to stand in the middle of the room. The facilitator will then explain that they will be asking 'would you rather' questions giving 2 options, each option will correlate to a side of the room. They will then ask 'would you rather ... or ...' giving 2 options that will correlate to a side of the room – the facilitator should point to the side of the room that each option correlates to.
b) Stand and sit – the facilitator should explain that they will be asking 'would you rather' questions giving 2 options, each option will correlate with either standing or sitting. The facilitator should then ask 'would you rather ... or ...' giving 2 options. They should inform the young people of which option correlates to standing or sitting.

Question ideas for would you rather:

- Film or TV series
- Rap or rock music
- Fight one horse sized duck or 50 duck sized horses

- McDonalds or KFC
- Football or basketball
- Have tongues for fingers or a finger for a tongue
- Hold a spider or a snake

Once facilitators have asked a few questions they may give young people the option to think of their own.

Skittles Game

Duration: 20–30 Minutes

Resources: Skittles

Each young person should be given a small amount of Skittles. The facilitator should explain each colour relates to a question. Attendees should be asked to choose 1–3 skittles; the number of skittles will depend on how much time is allocated for the activity, 1–3 skittles would mean the young people would be asked 1–3 questions.

If they have 2 skittles of the same colour, ask them to give an extra answer e.g. if they had 2 oranges – give their top 2 films.

Questions ideas for skittles game:

- Orange – What's your favourite film?
- Red – Something that makes you happy?
- Green – Something that winds you up?
- Yellow – A fun fact about you?
- Purple – Favourite food?

Questions can be adapted as needed. Young people may change the questions if they wish.

Human Bingo

Duration: 10 Minutes

Resources: Bingo sheets, pens

The young people will be given the example human bingo sheet, alternatively, facilitators may develop their own. The facilitator will ask the young people to find others in the group that relate to the description in the boxes (e.g. find someone who speaks a language). Once they have done this, they can write the person's name in the box. As far as possible, young people should try to have a different person in each box. However, if group size or other factors do not allow for this, the facilitator may set a limit of how many times one person can appear on the sheet.

Facilitators could tell the young people to aim for a line, the whole table, or both to win the bingo.

Flag of Me

Duration: 15–20 Minutes

Resources: Flag template, pens, pencils, colourful pens

Optional: Collage material, glue paint.

The young people will be given a template of a flag. The facilitator will explain that this flag will be to represent them. The young people can draw, write, stick, or paint anything that they feel represents them onto this flag. Some examples of prompts for the young people could be: What is important to them, what matters to them, things they like, what could they not live without (for example music, friends, books, singing, football, family)

The young people should be encouraged to share their flags with the group, explaining what they have included on their flag.

As an optional extra activity, the facilitator may ask the young people to pass their flags around the group and to add a comment on each other's flags. For example, if someone has written they like nature, another person may comment that they like nature too.

Energisers/Games

The following are short activities to aid re-engagement, particularly after a break.

Heads and Tails

Duration: 5 Minutes

Resources: Coin

The facilitator should explain that they will be playing heads and tails with a twist. The young people should be asked to stand and to choose heads or tails; if they choose heads, they put their hand on their head, if they choose tails, they put their hands on their tail bone.

The facilitator will flip a coin, whoever guessed correctly stays standing and plays the next round, whoever guessed wrong sits. The game keeps going until there is one person remaining, who is the winner.

Word Chain

Duration: 10 Minutes

Resources: N/A

The facilitator will decide on a word to start with, this will be a noun e.g. tree. The next person should say something that relates to the word tree, e.g. flower, the next person says something related to flower, e.g. grass. And so on, until someone gets stuck. This can then be started again with a new word.

References

1. Dressel, D.P. (2020). Breaking the Ice to Build Relationships: Using icebreakers to create new relationships, promote emotional safety, and incorporate social and emotional learning: Editor: Ferman Konukman. *Journal of Physical Education, Recreation & Dance*, *91*(5), 51–54.
2. Chlup, D.T., & Collins, T.E. (2010). Breaking the ice: Using ice-breakers and re-energizers with adult learners. *Adult Learning*, *21*(3–4), 34–39.
3. Zins, J.E., & Elias, M.J. (2007). Social and emotional learning: Promoting the development of all students. *Journal of Educational and Psychological Consultation*, *17*(2–3), 233–255.

7 Information Session

First Group Contact

Prior to delivering the psychometrics it is important to ensure that the attending young people have an understanding of the intervention. This provides an essential opportunity for facilitators to explain the intervention, address any questions and promote engagement. It may be useful to clarify to attendees that this session will not be the standard format for the intervention, and future sessions will be more interactive.

Some topics that should be covered in this session include:

- Purpose of the Intervention – explaining the aim and expected outcomes of the intervention, as described by this manual.
- Practical aspects – such as the expected duration of the program, the length of sessions and how breaks and holidays will be incorporated.
- The way of working of practitioners – highlighting the 'working together' values of the intervention and intention to support young people in their own goals.
- Safeguarding and Confidentiality – It is important for young people to be aware of the way information about them is recorded, how it is used and how it is kept safe (e.g. consent forms, how psychometrics are used). It is also essential for young people to understand the limits of confidentiality. This will promote openness, trust and allow young people to choose whether they want to make significant disclosures throughout the intervention. (See: 'Dealing with Difficult Issues' for more detail on breaking confidentiality)
- Data collection and use – If you are gathering data for the purposes of service evaluation, ensure participants and their carers are aware of how the data will be used in line with data protection regulations.

The delivery of this content can be aided by the 'SHERBET Information Leaflet for Young People' available in the resource section.

Facilitators should encourage questions at this point, to prevent unhelpful assumptions and beliefs about the program and to promote engagement.

It may be useful for facilitators to engage with the young people in a more casual way prior to the information session. This may involve sitting in their 'form time', chatting in the corridors or starting the session with an ice-breaker exercise. We have provided a variety of ice-breaker exercises within this manual for facilitators to use and adapt.

DOI: 10.4324/9781003666738-7

8 Individual Goal Planning Workshops

Individual interviews grant facilitators an opportunity to build rapport with young people and to gain a greater understanding of their needs and goals. It may also allow them to observe the young person's behaviour outside of a group setting. We have avoided the use of the word 'interview' with the young people when discussing these sessions. Young people are likely to have pre-existing expectations and fears surrounding interviews, particularly if they have experienced these within a social work or police setting. Referring to them as workshops prevents such associations and encourages young people to focus on the goal-setting task, rather than perceiving the session to be focusing on interrogating them.

Structure and Content of the Workshop

The following is a proposed structure for the individual interview/workshop with some suggested prompt questions. However, these may be adapted depending on the interview style of the facilitator and the responses of the young person. The important areas to cover are the themes to 'look out' for, as they provide essential knowledge about the young person's presenting problems, risk factors, protective factors, and motivations. These, in turn, will help facilitators tailor the approach during individual and group sessions.

Pre-group Workshop

This workshop is carried out prior to the start of the group. It primarily focuses on:

- Building rapport with attendees.
- Identifying any specific needs that would require adaptations in the group (e.g. Communication needs).
- Identifying relevant factors affecting the young person (e.g. triggers, motivations...).
- Identifying one main goal to support during sessions. This goal may not always be related to the young person's presenting problems, but facilitators should relate SHERBET content to it to improve engagement and motivation (e.g. If the young person wants a bike but their parents think they are not responsible enough for one, facilitators may highlight how SHERBET can help them manage their behaviour so they can show their parents that they are responsible).

DOI: 10.4324/9781003666738-8

Facilitators may also incorporate questions exploring risk and safeguarding concerns (e.g. suicide ideation, self-harm, at risk of victimisation) to ensure that the complexity and risk of attendees adheres to the requirements and capacity of facilitators and their organisations. Facilitators may then inform their approach with these responses (e.g. risk check-ins, safety plans), referring the young person to a more appropriate service if necessary.

Table 8.1

Duration Approx.	*Purpose and Sample Questions*	*Themes to 'look out' for*
5 min.	Introductions: Facilitators should introduce themselves and encourage the young person to do the same.	• Communication skills/ needs (preferred way of communicating). • Accessibility needs.
10 min.	Rapport Building: Facilitators may ask exploratory questions about the young person's life in order to find out relevant factors. This is also a good time to build rapport with the young person. Examples: - How long have you been in this school? - What subjects are you doing? - Do you have any plans/dreams for what to do after school? - Do you have any hobbies/work outside of school? - What do you do after school? - Tell me a bit about your typical day/weekend. - How do you get on with other students/teachers? - Tell me a bit about your friends/family… And any relevant 'tell me more about…' if the young person mentions something relevant.	• Instability in life (e.g. recent change in school). • Quality of Relationships (e.g. friendships, partners, teachers) and support systems. • Family relationships and dynamics. • Conflict with others. • Skills, goals, ambitions. • Relevant social pressures (class, gender, ethnicity, culture).
5 min.	Reaction to Information Session: Exploring what they have understood about the purpose of the intervention and how relevant it is to their needs and experiences in life. Do they recognise any problems? Examples: - What did you think of the information session on SHERBET? - Did you have any more questions about it? - Why do you think we've invited you to do SHERBET? - Do you think it could be useful for you? - Have you ever done a group like this before?	• Understanding of the Intervention. • Attitude towards the intervention. • Presenting Problems. • Insight into problems. • Emotion regulation difficulties. • Biases or beliefs that may hold them back. • Mental health needs.
10 min.	Goals Sheet: The end of the session should be dedicated to completing the 'Goal-setting' worksheet in collaboration with the young person. This may not all be completed within the time but at least the final 'step' of the goal and the 'where am I now' should be completed. Any links between the goal and the intervention should be highlighted, to highlight the collaborative nature of SHERBET and promote engagement and adherence.	• Motivations. • Engagement. • How the goal may relate to the program?

Post-group Workshop

This workshop is carried out after the end of the group sessions. It primarily focuses on:

- Exploring the young person's progress with their presenting difficulties and their 'main goal' identified in the pre-group workshop.
- Assessing the young person's remaining needs.
- Planning for adequate support after the end of the group (e.g. re-referral, closing the case, sharing resources with school staff and family...).
- Highlighting positive progress to maintain motivation and adherence to the skills and knowledge obtained.
- Seeking feedback for their experience of SHERBET.

Facilitators may also incorporate questions exploring risk and safeguarding concerns (e.g. suicide ideation, self-harm, at risk of victimisation...) to inform their recommendations (e.g. referral to further support).

Table 8.2

Duration Approx.	*Purpose and Sample Questions*	*Themes to 'look out' for*
5 min.	Check-in: Facilitators should begin the session with a general wellbeing check-in. In this way facilitators may support students to feel comfortable. This check-in may also identify relevant worries or challenges which facilitators need to address to improve engagement prior to proceeding with the workshop. Examples: - How have you been? - How was school today? Facilitators may also ask about something which the young person has previously mentioned or shown interest in (e.g. you mentioned you had a match yesterday, how did it go?)	• Worries or challenges which may require support before continuing the workshop.
5 min.	Progress with Problems and Goals: Facilitators should review the Goals Worksheet with attendees and inquire about their progress within this. Some attendees may struggle to identify and accept positive change. Facilitators may support young people by sharing times that they observed positive change in the young person. Examples: - What was your main goal when joining the group? - How close are you to achieving this goal (1–10)? - Do you feel you have made progress towards this goal? Why/why not? And any relevant 'tell me more about…' if the young person mentions something relevant.	• Motivations. • Engagement. • Insight into their problems. • Insight into their progress.

(*Continued*)

Table 8.2 (Continued)

Duration Approx.	*Purpose and Sample Questions*	*Themes to 'look out' for*
5 min.	Helpful skills and protective factors: Facilitators may proceed by exploring what factors were helpful to the young people. These may include elements from inside and outside the group. Examples: - What do you think has helped you get closer to your goals? Why/how? - What things in SHERBET did you find most helpful? Why? - Has anything happened outside of SHERBET that has also been helpful? - What are some things you have learned that you do not want to forget?	• Understanding of the Intervention. • Attitude towards the intervention. • Protective factors. • Helpful tools and skills.
5 min.	Feedback on SHERBET: Facilitators should explore areas of improvement for SHERBET. These may also provide valuable information for schools (e.g. by highlighting things that attendees find helpful/unhelpful in lessons). Facilitators should reassure attendees that negative feedback is welcomed and will not have an impact on attendees. Example: - What is something you did not like about SHERBET? - Was there anything you would change about our sessions to make them better? - What was your favourite session? Why?	• Potential triggers or unhelpful approaches for the young person.
10 min.	Future Planning: Facilitators should explore any remaining needs and difficulties for the young person. Facilitators may then share options for what to do next (e.g. closure, new referral, continue to support 1:1...) and collaboratively plan next steps with attendees. - You mentioned you still struggle with X, do you need more support with this? - You have certainly achieved a lot within the group, are there any things you still want to work on or need help with? - What kind of help do you think might be useful? What things would you like to do or learn? If no further support is needed at present, facilitators should ensure students are aware of who they may speak to if their difficulties return (e.g. for support or re-referral).	• Remaining Problems. • Mental health problems. • Need for further support.

Workshop Delivery Style

Individual interviews, as well as the format of delivery of the whole intervention, should be underpinned by a motivational and compassionate approach. Although not all facilitators will have formal training on Motivational Interviewing, awareness of their purpose and the inclusion of related strategies is encouraged.

Motivational Interviewing (MI): Further guidance may be found at motivationalinterviewing.org

> *MI is a collaborative, goal-oriented style of communication with particular attention to the language of change. It is designed to strengthen personal motivation for and commitment to a specific goal by eliciting and exploring the person's own reasons for change within an atmosphere of acceptance and compassion.*
>
> *Miller & Rollnick, 2013, p. 29*[1]

Key qualities include[1, 2]:

- Facilitators should engage as equal partners with the young people, using active listening skills and refraining from unsolicited advice, confronting, instructing, directing, or warning.
- MI is designed to guide and empower people to change by eliciting their own meaning, motivation and capacity for change.
- MI is based on respect and curiosity as guides for communication and exploration. It aims to facilitate change, whilst respecting client autonomy.

Some Core Skills include[1, 2]:

- Using **Open questions**. These may focus on the person's experiences and beliefs. Open questions guide clients to reflect on how change may be achievable whilst preventing facilitators from asserting a 'right answer'.
  Open questions may also be used as a strategy to offer information. This can be done by exploring what the person has shared or already knows, seeking permission for the practitioner to share information, followed by an exploration of what the client thinks of this. (e.g. 'You were saying... That makes me think... What do you think?)
- Using **Affirmations** and praise of client strengths, efforts and previous achievements. This aims to build the client's hope, self-esteem, and self-efficacy so they can feel confident in their ability to change.
- **Reflections** such as repeating, rephrasing, or offering a deeper exploration about what the person is trying to communicate. These reflections aim to obtain a deeper understanding of the client and showcase that the facilitator is listening and is invested in understanding.
- **Summarizing** promotes shared understanding and highlights key points made by the client.
- **Collaborative working** honours that both the facilitator and client have expertise. Discussions and information sharing within MI is considered a two-way street and the experiential expertise of clients should be acknowledged and valued.

Stages of Change

MI uses the Stages of Change model[3] to guide and track behavioural changes. Recognising where a client is in their process of change can aid practitioners in identifying what strategies will be most effective to guide their progress.[1–4] The stages include:

- Precontemplation: The person is not seeking change or is unaware of the need to change. They may be denying or unaware of problems.
  MI Advises: Encourage the client to reflect on their behaviour. Increase ambivalence by exploring the negative impacts of the behaviour and reflecting these back in conversation. Increase awareness of the problem.
- Contemplation: The person now recognises there is a problem and is considering change, but they're unsure or uncertain about change.
  MI Advises: Support the client to explore and compare their options, including the benefits and challenges of change.
- Preparation: The person recognises the problem, is committed to change, and is making specific plans to achieve change.
  MI Advises: Support the client to develop a specific plan, based on realistic goals and accounting for relevant barriers. Build the client's confidence in their ability to adhere to the plan.
- Action: The person is acting upon plans, engaging in behaviours that align with the change they seek. They are actively working towards their goals.
  MI Advises: Support the client by providing encouragement and feedback as they proceed with their plan. Support them to adapt their plan as necessary if unforeseen barriers arise.
- Maintenance: The person has successfully engaged in the action stage and has now maintained behaviour change for a period of time. Adhering to the changed behaviour is potentially less effortful than in the action stage. The person is working to prevent relapse.
  MI Advises: Support the client to strengthen their skills so they may maintain their progress long-term: Building resilience and strategies for barriers and challenges that they anticipate. Praise and reinforce their progress.
- Relapse: The person returns to old behaviours.
  MI Advises: Help the client reflect. Learn from the relapse and re-engage in the change process. Clients may experience shame and hopelessness that will hold them back from re-engaging. Help re-build confidence and hope.

It is important to understand that individuals will cycle through these changes, and relapses in behaviour are part of this cycle. Each cycle through the stages of change, including relapse, is an opportunity for learning and reflection. It can be challenging for both staff and clients to maintain hope and confidence when facing barriers and relapses. Understanding the process of change can help staff recognise where clients are in their journey, guiding them in how to provide the most effective support.

Adapting to a Group – Group Goal Planning Workshop

It may be that constraints exist that do not permit facilitators to conduct an individual goal planning workshop with each child. Facilitators may not have the time due to their overall caseload, schools may not have the facilities or the staff to support the process, young people may struggle to engage on a 1:1 format...

Evidence for the comparison of effectiveness between group and individual MI interventions is limited.[5] Initial research suggested that a group is not as effective as individual delivery and a blended approach was recommended, although differences were not significant.[5] However, more recent evidence has suggested that MI groups are effective in supporting treatment engagement and completion, building insight into problems and increasing perceived autonomy, preparedness to change and self-efficacy.[6]

Overall, it is preferred that the Goal Planning Workshop is delivered individually. However, it is appropriate for this to be adapted to a group delivery if practical constraints are present. Adaptations may also be made to improve the efficacy of group approaches.[7, 8]

When delivering a group Goal Planning Workshop, facilitators will have to pay particular attention to group interactions. Member feedback may sometimes come across as judgemental, critical, or self-interested rather than empathetic and motivational. Facilitators should endeavour to promote mutual respect and collaboration amongst attendees, model positive ways of providing feedback, and gently redirect less helpful comments and responses. The redirection of unhelpful comments may be done by:

- Reframing unhelpful contributions.
- Reminding the group of the guidelines (e.g. respect, not criticising...).
- Returning to an appropriate conversation, potentially asking the original commenter (or another group member if they struggle) to reframe their comment or question.

Facilitators may also maintain an individualised and tailored focus, whilst ensuring that group discussions are relevant to all attendees, by blending individual and group processes. There are multiple methods to manage this:

- Facilitators may focus on different attendees at different points of the session, with brief but focused individual conversations. They may then use open-ended questions to generalise discussions to the larger group. For example, 'Who else is feeling/ experiencing … (Insert theme of the interaction e.g. powerlessness, conflict...)?'
  By focusing on themes and feelings facilitators can emphasise similarities across the group, supporting cohesiveness and support across attendees.
- Facilitators may assign time for attendees to work individually on their goals worksheets. They may then engage in conversations with individual attendees, addressing specific needs which may differ from the group or which they may be reluctant to share in group discussion. This is an appropriate time to focus on specific practical aspects of the goals, as these are likely to be highly individual to each attendee and their goal.

References

1 Miller, W.R., & Rollnick, S. (2013). *Motivational interviewing: Helping people to change* (3rd ed.). Guilford Press.

2 Miller, W.R., & Moyers, T.B. (2017). Motivational interviewing and the clinical science of Carl Rogers. *Journal of Consulting and Clinical Psychology, 85*(8), 757–766.

3 Prochaska, J.O., & DiClemente, C.C. (1983). Stages and processes of self-change of smoking: Toward an integrative model of change. *Journal of Consulting and Clinical Psychology, 51*(3), 390–395.

4 Zimmerman, G.L., Olsen, C.G., & Bosworth, M.F. (2000). A 'stages of change' approach to helping patients change behavior. *American Family Physician, 61*(5), 1409–1416.

5 Lundahl, B.W., Kunz, C., Brownell, C., Tollefson, D., & Burke, B.L. (2010). A meta-analysis of motivational interviewing: Twenty-five years of empirical studies. *Research on Social Work Practice*, *20*(2), 137–160.

6 Wagner, C.C., & Ingersoll, K.S. (2012). *Motivational interviewing in groups*. Guilford Press.

7 Velasquez, M.M., Stephens, N.S., & Ingersoll, K. (2006). Motivational interviewing in groups. *Journal of Groups in Addiction & Recovery*, *1*(1), 27–50.

8 Krejci, J., & Neugebauer, Q. (2015). Motivational interviewing in groups: Group process considerations. *Journal of Groups in Addiction & Recovery*, *10*(1), 23–40.

9 Session 1

Getting Started

Task 1: Introductions

Duration: *10 Minutes (+ Icebreaker duration)*
Objectives: *Build Rapport with attendees*
Group Interaction
Reinforcing knowledge and understanding about the program
Resources: *SHERBET Leaflets for Children and Young People*
Icebreaker Task

Facilitators may have already introduced themselves and the program during the psychometrics group session. Nonetheless, they should allocate some time to review the information and answer any questions from the young people.

This may be supplemented by the use of an ice-breaker task, which can be used to build rapport with the young people. Please refer to our Icebreaker section for a selection of tasks. Some particularly useful icebreakers for each session may include:

- Brief introductions including name and pronouns
- Which 'Mood' are you today?
- What's your favourite ...?
- Skittles game
- 2 truths 1 lie

Task 2: Group Agreements

Duration: *15 Minutes*
Objectives: *Building Boundaries*
Group Interaction
Promoting young people's investment and ownership of the group
Generating a safe space for young people
Resources: *Whiteboard OR Flipchart paper AND pens to write with*

Group agreements, or group rules, should be collaboratively developed by facilitators and young people. Facilitators should set up a board or piece of paper that all the young people can see.

Facilitators will explain that the host organisation already has some rules to keep everyone safe, and these still apply within the group. However, within the group we want to get their own

DOI: 10.4324/9781003666738-9

opinions on what guidelines would be useful so that the sessions can be safe and respectful and comfortable.

A good example to begin with is 'respect each other' – facilitators should encourage young people to share what respect means to them and be specific about which behaviours can show respect. Good examples may include: Listen when someone else is talking, use kind language towards each other...

This may be a good time to review the confidentiality guidelines. Facilitators should ensure that young people are aware of the situations in which they would have to break confidentiality. It may also be appropriate to discuss with young people how they would like to be informed if confidentiality needs to be broken e.g. told by facilitators before passing on the information (when appropriate and safe to do so), told by teachers etc.

Be open to creativity and adapting to the specific needs of the group. Some groups may benefit from having a 'time out' sign which they can use when feeling overwhelmed so they can step out of the room. Some groups may choose to have shorter breaks more often, rather than a longer break mid-session. The availability and use of sensory toys may also be included in the group agreements.

Overall, this exercise hopes to promote collaborative working with young people. It shows them that their opinions and choices are respected. Feeling ownership over the group functioning may also promote adherence to the program and rules themselves, as rules that 'don't make sense' have been shown to negatively impact young people's mood, behaviour, and treatment adherence.[1]

Task 3: The World Around Us

Duration: *30 Minutes*
Objectives: *Group Interaction*
Learning about the Social-Ecological Model[2, 3]
Learning about the 'Circles of Control' Theory[4]
Gaining an understanding about Young People's environment and Influences
Resources: *Ecological Model Worksheet*
Whiteboard OR Flipchart paper AND pens to write with
Pens for the Young People

Facilitators may print out a large version of the Ecological Model or draw it on an available board/flipchart paper. They can then provide brief definitions for each of the 'circles' within the model (It may also be appropriate to give one example for each circle):

Individual circle (Child)	The person themselves! Their choices and actions. May also include biological and personal history factors.
Relationship circle (Microsystem)	Close relationships and influences that have direct contact with the child. E.g. Friends
Community circle (Mesosystem)	The settings, such as schools, workplaces, and neighbourhoods, in which relationships take place.
Society circle (Macrosystem)	Societal factors such as policies, social and cultural norms.

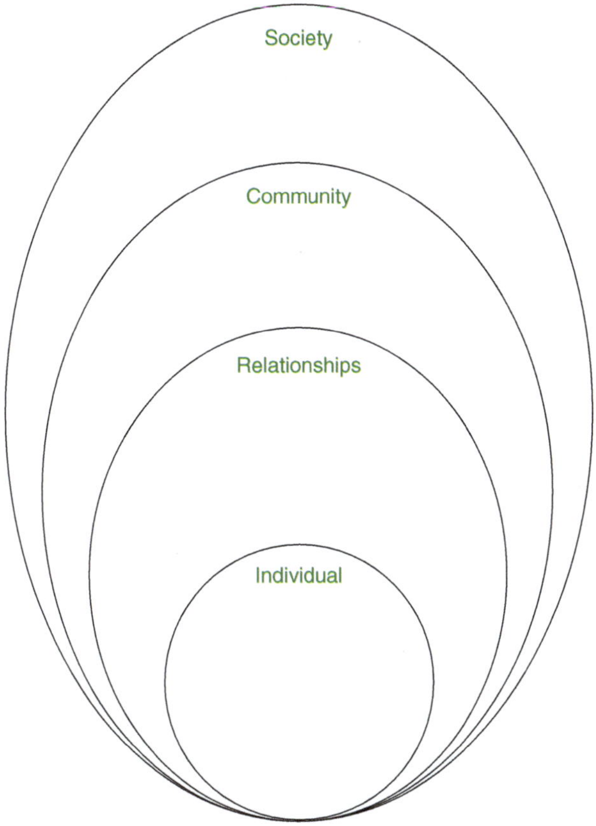

Figure 9.1

We have provided a list of possible influences which the young people, as a group, can sort into the appropriate circles within the sample model. By completing a generic sample model as a group, young people should build understanding of the different systems, their definitions and examples. This will equip them for the next step of the exercise, which is applying these models to their own life and experience.

We have provided a **resource sheet** with visual and written prompts. Facilitators may print and cut this sheet to support young people with this exercise. The examples of influences may be presented one at a time for young people to consider and sort as needed.

Relevant 'Circle'	*Examples of Influences*
Society	History Culture Laws Mass Media (TV, newspapers, news websites)

Relevant 'Circle'	*Examples of Influences*
Community	Extended Family (Some children may place this in 'relationships' if they are close with their extended family) School Social Media Neighbourhood
Relationships	Siblings Parents Friends Girlfriend/Boyfriend/Partner
Individual	Knowledge Personality Mental Health

Following this, **young people can fill in their own worksheets ('The World Around Us' section)** with the influences which are applicable to them – these may vary depending on who is in their lives and the weight they give to their influence! Facilitators should encourage young people to tailor their worksheet to their own individual experience, adding their own 'influences' on their circles as opposed to just using the examples provided. This will allow for a more tailored and in-depth insight. As they complete the worksheets, young people can be encouraged to discuss these influences: How much do they affect them (label them on a 1–10 scale)? Are they positive or negative?

After completing the worksheet facilitators may move onto the 'Influencing Life' section of the worksheet (which covers the 'circles of influence' theory). Young people will be prompted to reflect on how much control and influence they have over different areas of their lives.
We need to focus our energies on what we can control and influence!

1. *CIRCLE OF CONTROL: what we can directly control.*
2. *CIRCLE OF INFLUENCE: The worries that we can do something about.*
3. *CIRCLE OF CONCERN: Wide range of worries which we cannot change right now.*

Facilitators may increase the interactive nature of the activity by asking young people to stand in different areas of the room if they think a certain item is part of their circle of control, influence, or concern. Prompts may include the influences discussed in the 'Ecological Model' (e.g. mental health, family, laws...). These prompts should be read one at a time, giving young people sufficient time to move around the room safely (e.g. no running). Once they have selected their answer, young people may be asked to explain their choice.

Young people should be encouraged to reflect that they mainly have control over themselves and their choices. They may be able to influence some areas and people to an extent, but there will be factors out of their full control.

Some examples may be used to illustrate this concept: A young person may want to encourage their friend to join the same activities as them. They may be able to convince and influence their friend but, at the end of the day, it is their friend's choice, and they can't fully control it. The same can be said the other way around. Others may try to influence or provoke them, but they have the control over their own reactions and behaviours.

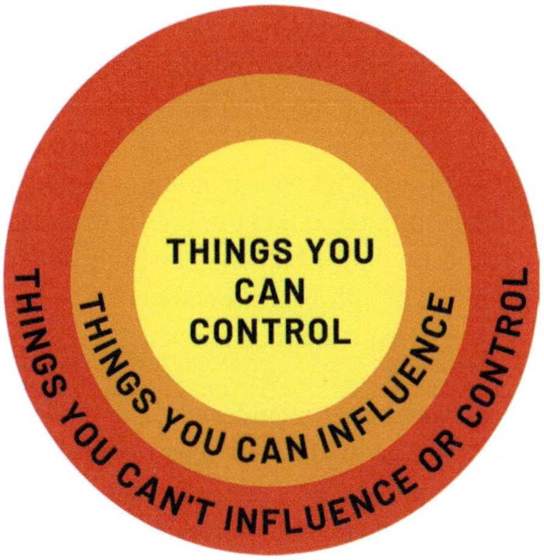

Figure 9.2

Facilitators may link this back to the focus of the group – during sessions we will think about the challenges that the world brings us, but we will always bring it back to the young person's control over their choices and actions. During sessions facilitators can also return to the concept of 'circles of control' to challenge young people's worries and concerns about areas which are out of their control ('circle of concern') and may be more beneficial to let go of.

Extension Activity: Prompt young people to think of how they feel when they cannot control something in their environment. How do they react to it?

Task 4: My Coat of Arms

Duration: *15 Minutes*
Objectives: *Group Interaction, building group relationships*
Building Attendees' Self-efficacy
Resources: *Coat of Arms Worksheets*
Pens for the Young People

This task aims to highlight to attendees how the content covered throughout the goals workshop and first session relates to them. It also aims to promote self-efficacy (i.e. the belief that they can successfully achieve their goals) by encouraging young people to think of strengths in themselves and their environment.

The 'coat of arms' contains five sections. Young people are encouraged to fill in each of their sections, by writing or drawing:

- A little about me: Write or draw your name and a little about yourself. For example:
  - Favourite food
  - Favourite colour
  - If you have any pets
- Something that brings me joy: Write or draw something or someone that makes you feel happy. It does not have to be big or exciting, the 'little things in life' also count!

- Something I like about myself: Write or draw something about yourself that makes you feel happy or proud. Think about your personality, achievements, skills...
- Something good in my world: We have explored 'the world around us' in this session. Write or draw about something or someone who is a good influence in your life. Why do they make your life better?
- Something I can overcome: It would not be a coat of arms without winning a battle! Write or draw about a challenge that you will face in the group (e.g. talking in public, making new friends...)? Then, have a little think about how you can win the battle against this challenge. *Hint: We are stronger together! Share your challenge with other members of the group. Maybe they have ideas on how you can win the battle, or even ideas on how they can help you!

These sections and descriptions are included in the worksheet for attendees.

It is important for facilitators to promote variety in the coat of arms, so that as many strengths as possible may be identified. For example, if a young person says that what they like about themselves is their skills at sport, facilitators should encourage them to think of something other than sport for 'something that brings me joy'.

Once attendees have added adequate detail to their coat of arms these may be discussed in a group setting. In particular, facilitators should encourage group collaboration for 'something I can overcome'. Young people should be encouraged to give each other advice and support, promoting a collaborative approach for future sessions.

Task 5: Homework

Duration: *5–10 Minutes*
Objectives: *Promoting youth involvement*
Planning for the next session
Resources: *Whiteboard OR Flipchart paper AND pens to write with*

If possible, facilitators should carry out this task at the end of session 1. If this is not possible due to time constraints, this can be given out as a homework task for young people to bring in session 2.

Staff should explain that in session 2 we will be playing different songs and thinking about how they show different emotions (anger, stress, love, sadness, happiness, etc) or bring up emotions in us. Young people should then be asked to think about songs which they think would be good for this task.

Young people may then suggests different songs. They should avoid saying which emotion they link the song to (as this task will be done next week and we don't want to influence peers' interpretations of the songs).

Facilitators can make a note of these suggestions and prepare them for next session. Facilitators should review the songs to ensure that they are appropriate for the age group taking part in the session.

References

1 Gros, C.P., Parr, C., Wright, D.K., Montreuil, M., & Frechette, J. (2017). Hospital rules and regulations: The perspectives of youth receiving psychiatric care. *Journal of Child and Adolescent Psychiatric Nursing*, *30*(1), 18–24.

2 Bronfenbrenner, U. (1992). *Ecological systems theory*. Jessica Kingsley Publishers.
3 Krug, E.G., Mercy, J.A., Dahlberg, L.L., & Zwi, A.B. (2002). The world report on violence and health. *The Lancet*, *360*(9339), 1083–1088.
4 Covey, S.R. (2004). *The 7 habits of highly effective people: Powerful lessons in personal change*. Simon and Schuster.

10 Session 2

Recognising Emotions in Ourselves

Task 1: Emotion Wheel

Duration: *15–20 Minutes (+ Icebreaker duration)*
Objectives: *Build Rapport with attendees*
Group Interaction
Explore existing knowledge about emotions
Resources: *Whiteboard OR Flipchart paper AND pens to write with*
Emotion Wheel Worksheet

This task may be preceded by a check-in or icebreaker task.
Facilitators should encourage young people to shout out the names of as many emotions as they can think of. If there are quiet members in the group, this is an easy and ideal exercise to encourage their involvement. Maybe ask young people to go around the room in order, to ensure that all young people get a chance to speak. Facilitators may give young people some thinking time before sharing their responses.

Facilitators can write all the suggestions onto the white-board or flipchart paper as they are called out. After approximately 5 minutes, facilitators can end the suggestions round. Facilitators may then provide the following facts:

- How many different emotions can a human experience? (Get young people to guess an answer!)

A recent study by UC Berkeley[1] concluded that there are 27 basic human emotions. If we calculate out all possible combinations of 27 we get the number

134 MILLION.

That is a lot! No wonder people can feel overwhelmed, lost, and confused when it comes to feeling, recognising, and talking about emotions.

Facilitators may then bring out the **emotion wheel worksheets**. Staff can explain that emotion wheels have been used to help people of all ages gain knowledge and skills surrounding emotions.

Facilitators should give young people a few minutes to familiarise themselves with the tool. Some useful discussion points may include:

- How do you think the emotion wheel is used? How can we use it in sessions?

DOI: 10.4324/9781003666738-10

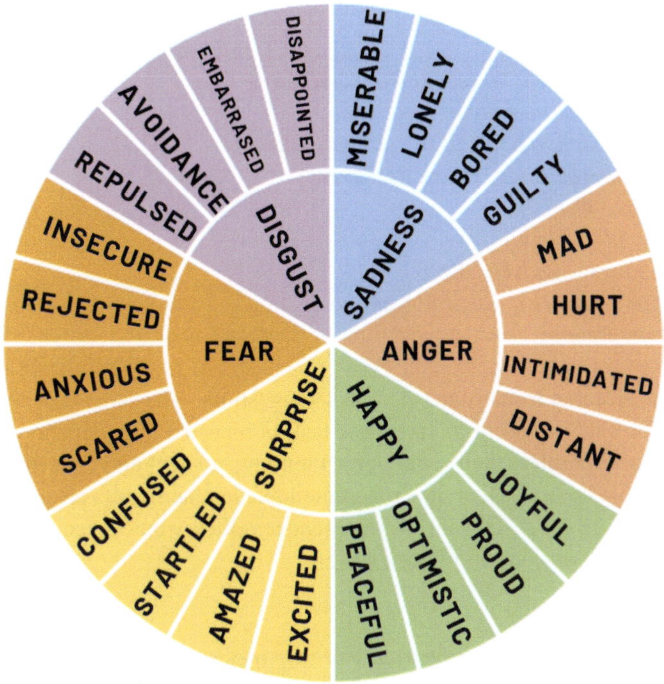

Figure 10.1

Emotion wheels are a teaching and communication tool. They help us learn the names of different emotions. The way that they are laid out also makes it easy to find the word for more complex emotions (e.g. between sad and angry or between happy and surprised). Emotion wheels can also be used when we feel lost or overwhelmed. Sometimes talking about emotions can be hard, and we can't get the help we need because we can't explain how we are feeling. We can use an emotion wheel to simply point at how we are feeling if we are struggling to use our words.

- Are there any emotions on the wheel that have new or unfamiliar names? Can anyone else describe or define them? (if no young people can define them, facilitators may provide an answer).

Young people may notice that this tool does not have 27 emotions in its centre, it only has 6 (Fear, Sadness, Disgust, Anger, Surprise, and Happy). We thought 27 might be a bit much to start with, so we are keeping things simple and following the model by Ekman (1992).[2] One other place where they may have seen some of these emotions might be the 2015 film, Inside Out – discuss it if appropriate!

Task 2: Mapping Emotions

Duration: *50 Minutes*
Objectives: *Explore young people's skills in recognising emotions*
Explore the valence and intensity of emotions
Practicing 'coming back to neutral' (i.e. calming down)
Resources: *'Physical Emotion in the Body' Visual Resource*
'Mapping Emotions' Worksheet
Set of Speakers to play music
Prepared list of songs (and lyric sheets)
Software to access music (e.g. Spotify, Youtube...)
Pens for the Young People

Songs from this task may be selected from young people's suggestions. The same task will be repeated for different emotions. The amount of times the task is repeated may depend on the speed with which young people complete their reflections, their engagement and concentration on the task and the time available in the session. It is recommended that facilitators prioritise the exploration of emotions which are most relevant to the attendees (they would have identified these from the referrals and initial sessions and interviews).

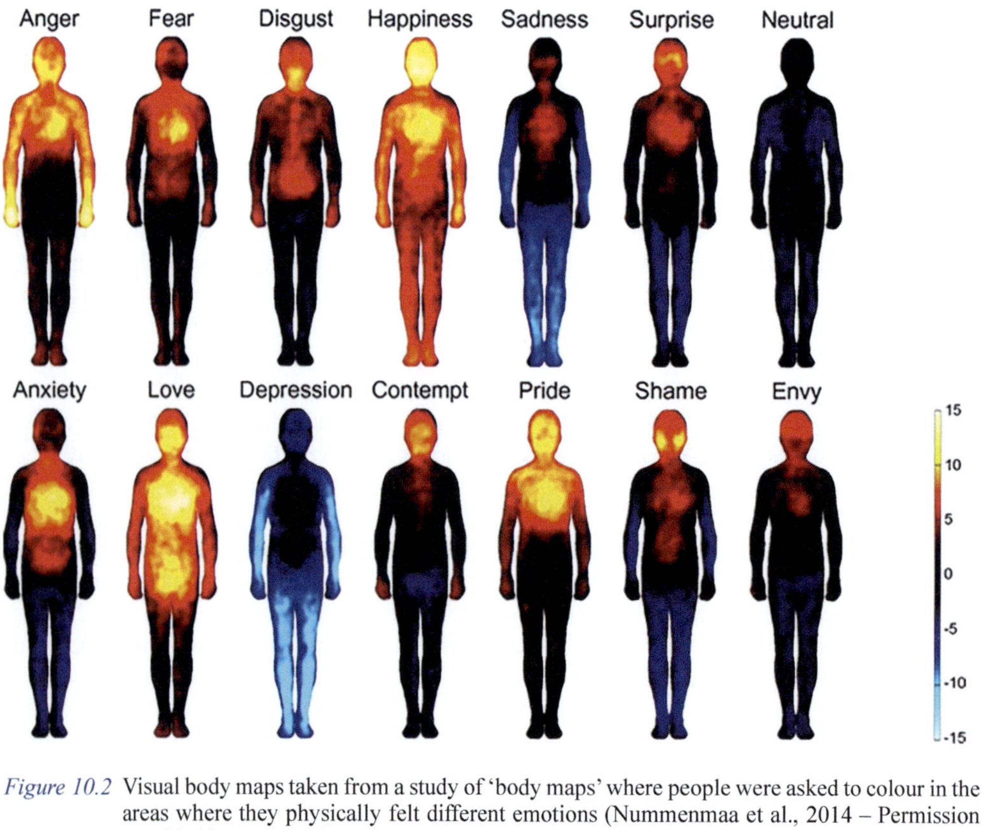

Figure 10.2 Visual body maps taken from a study of 'body maps' where people were asked to colour in the areas where they physically felt different emotions (Nummenmaa et al., 2014 – Permission provided by study authors).

Prior to beginning the task, facilitators should explain to young people the content of the worksheet and how the task will work.

This may be assisted by the 'Physical emotion in the Body' Visual Resource (See Right) – This resource is taken from a study of 'body maps' where people were asked to colour in the areas where they physically felt different emotions[3] (e.g. chest tightness, feeling a pit in your stomach, feeling butterflies...). It is worth being aware that these examples are the combination of hundreds of different people's body maps. There are areas that we have in common, but we may also have differences – that is normal and expected! Young people should be reminded that there are no right or wrong answers in these exercises.

The task structure is as follows:

1. Play the song of choice (or a selected portion): Facilitators should already have awareness of the content and appropriateness of the song, as well as some awareness of which emotions it may elicit. If possible, facilitators should provide the lyrics to the song so attendees may refer to them (e.g. using a printout, screen, or projector)
2. As the song plays, young people should colour in their body map. Attendees may use different colours depending on whether they perceive the emotions as positive or negative, or use written labels. They should also make a note of how intense the emotion feels (e.g. on a scale of 1–10). Facilitators are welcome to join in with their own worksheets.
3. After the music has stopped, young people and facilitators may compare and discuss their body maps and ratings. It is expected that there will be differences.
   Facilitators should prompt young people to use their words to explain their drawings and ratings (e.g. Why did you colour X? What was the sensation? What makes you give it that rating of intensity out of 10? How would it feel if it was higher?). Facilitators may model responses by describing their own charts.
   Young people may be encouraged to name the emotion they felt (with help of the emotion wheel if needed) – different people may feel different emotions and different intensities as the result of a same song!
4. Explore the functions of the emotion (or emotions if more than one has been identified) that the song has elicited. Are these functions helpful or unhelpful? Examples of functions may include[4, 5]:

Information: Emotions can tell us a lot about our environment. Surprise tells us that there is new information we were not aware before. Anger, fear or discomfort tell us that something may be wrong, and we need to look out for it or fix it. Disgust can tell us when food may be unsafe, so we don't get sick!

Downside – Sometimes emotions can distract and 'cloud' our judgement so that we see the world through that emotion. Think of how love may give you 'rose tinted glasses' or how fear may make us think that safe situations are dangerous (e.g. anxiety).

Communication: Emotions can help us communicate with others. By empathising with others, we may feel how they are feeling – this can help us understand them and build better relationships. Knowing our emotions can also help us communicate (we will look at this in later sessions!).

Downside – Again, emotions can be very influential and may negatively impact our communication if they become very intense! Think – Could you have a calm conversation when you're very angry? Is it sometimes hard to talk when you're very upset? Is it hard to stay on topic when you're very excited about something?

Call to Action: Happiness, Anger, and Fear can be very powerful energisers – they give us energy to do actions. For example: Anger and Fear were useful to keep us safe in the past, when we may have had to 'Fight' or 'Flight' predators. Happiness and determination can help us do tasks which we like or are good for us.

Downside – Extreme emotions can sometimes give us too much energy at inappropriate times. As a result, we may behave in ways that we don't like, or which hurt others or ourselves. For example, have you ever shouted at someone you care about just because you were angry at the time? Have you ever felt like punching something or someone even though you know that would not be a good thing to do?

Pleasantness: Some emotions can feel very nice! Calm, happiness, love...

Downside – Sometimes we can become a bit obsessed with achieving these pleasant feelings, to the point where we're almost 'hooked' to certain behaviours. Think of people who take substances so they can feel calm or happy, people who are constantly in relationships with bad people to avoid feeling unpleasant loneliness... Or even the focus a lot of us have on achieving 'happiness' in life, to the point that people get very stressed and obsessed with this goal!

Call to Stop: Emotions can help us stop unhelpful behaviours. Fear can make us 'freeze' in the moment, this used to be an advantageous behaviour to keep us safe, but its usefulness can vary. Disgust and fear can help us avoid dangerous situations. Calmness can help us stop and think before acting.
Downside – Intense fear, anger, and sadness can lead us to 'freezing' or hiding away from other people. This can stop us from communicating and getting help when we need it.

5. After the emotion has been adequately explored, before moving onto the next song, young people will be encouraged to 'return to neutral'. In order to not muddle the emotions of one song and another (similar to a pallet cleanser) young people will be encouraged to take part in a breathing and relaxation exercise or listening to a 'calming' song so that they can return to a neutral state before tackling the next song. This may be supported using the 'deep breathing' leaflet, which provides a guide to different deep breathing exercises.

Song Suggestions

Emotion	*Song Title*	*Artist*	*Timestamp Reference (YouTube)*
Anger	Seventeen Going Under	Sam Fender	1.10 – 2.37
	Good 4 U	Olivia Rodrigo	0.22 – 1.09
	Big for your Boots	Stormzy	0.00 – 1.00
Sadness	I hate U I love U	Gnash	0.00 – 1.00
	Carry me Home	Jorja Smith	0.00 – 1.00
	Memories	Maroon 5	0.00 – 0.32

Emotion	*Song Title*	*Artist*	*Timestamp Reference (YouTube)*
Happiness	Sunday Best	Surfaces	0.30 – 1.35
	On the Low	Burna Boy	00.10 – 01:00
	Uptown Funk	Bruno Mars	00.10 – 1:30
Fear	Mother Mother	Hayloft	1.00 – 1.20
Calm	Caribbean Blue	Enya	0.05 – 1.00
	Put Your Records On	Ritt Momney	0.00 – 1.14
	Ghost Choir	Louie Zong	0.00 – 1.29

Task 3: Homework Task – Relaxation Playlist

Duration: 5 Minutes
Objectives: Practice relaxation using calming music
Resources: Software to access music (e.g. Spotify, Youtube...)

Facilitators may set a homework task for the young people to complete in between sessions. Young people may be encouraged to apply the skills they have learned in this session by creating a relaxation playlist. Young people should create a playlist with songs that help them feel calm. When they listen to the playlist they should check in with their body – does this song make their body feel calm and relaxed?

The relaxation playlist is a tool that young people may continue to use between sessions to practice their relaxation skills.

References

1 Cowen, A.S., & Keltner, D. (2017). Self-report captures 27 distinct categories of emotion bridged by continuous gradients. *Proceedings of the National Academy of Sciences, 114*(38), E7900–E7909.

2 Ekman, P. (1992). Facial expressions of emotion: New findings, new questions. *Psychological Science, 3*(1), 34–38

3 Nummenmaa, L., Glerean, E., Hari, R., & Hietanen, J.K. (2014). Bodily maps of emotions. *Proceedings of the National Academy of Sciences, 111*(2), 646–651.

4 Hwang, H., & Matsumoto, D. (2019). "Functions of emotions". In *Noba textbook series: Psychology*, edited by R. Biswas-Diener and E. Diener. DEF Publishers. https://nobaproject.com/modules/functi ons-of-emotions

5 Newman, B.M., & Newman, P.R. (2017). *Development through life: A psychosocial approach.* Cengage Learning.

11 Session 3

Recognising Emotions in Ourselves (Part 2)

Task 1: Check-In

Duration: *10 Minutes (+ Icebreaker duration)*
Objectives: *Promote peer support and reflection*
Explore attendee knowledge retention
Resources: *None*
This task may be preceded by an icebreaker task.

Facilitators may benefit from reviewing attendee's retention of the information covered in session 1. Facilitators can provide visual prompts (e.g. blank 'mapping emotions' worksheet) and ask attendees to explain what they did and why it was important. Some other relevant prompts include:

- Tell me one thing you remember from last week.
- Can you name one positive/negative function of anger (or another emotion)?
- How confident did people feel in labelling the emotion and intensity level? Is this easier to do than before session 2?

Facilitators may also benefit from checking in with attendee attitudes and wellbeing at the beginning of the session, as these are likely to impact their engagement throughout. By identifying and addressing these needs early in the session, facilitators may increase the quality and quantity of engagement.

Task 2: Emotion Thermometer

Duration: *50 Minutes*
Objectives: *Continue developing skills in recognising emotions*
Exploring the intensity of emotions and how they affect us
Practicing 'coming back to neutral' (i.e. calming down)
Resources: *'Emotion Thermometer' Worksheet*

Information for Facilitators

This exercise aims to create 'Emotion Thermometers'. These focus on the main emotion which is causing difficulty for each attendee (e.g. anger, stress, fear), and explore how the emotion

DOI: 10.4324/9781003666738-11

presents itself at different levels of intensity (e.g. warning signs, behaviours...). It also explores potentially helpful strategies, matching them to the level of intensity where they would be most effective (e.g. attempting to explain their feelings may not be feasible at a 10/10 intensity of anger).

This worksheet, once completed, aims to fulfil the role of a Positive Behaviour Support (PBS) plan.[1]

PBS Plans have been effective in supporting people with challenging behaviours (e.g. aggression, self-harm...), even presentations which were considered severe and high-rate.[2, 3] Instead of focusing on punishment, PBS Plans aim to prevent the unhelpful behaviour from happening by avoiding unnecessary triggers and building helpful skills and alternative behaviours.[1] PBS is, in origin, an overarching service model and is therefore most effective if it is widely and consistently implemented within a person's life (e.g. school, home, etc.).[1, 4]

The present worksheet includes multiple PBS elements:

- It is person-centred (considers the needs and goals of the child).
- It considers the function of the child's behaviour (What are they trying to achieve?).
- It considers mediator variables (e.g. triggers, rewards... External elements that may impact the behaviour).
- It includes strategies which the young person can do alone and accompanied, as well as strategies that third parties may use to support the young person.
- It includes strategies at 3 levels. Examples for each level have been provided for both child-led and third party-led strategies.

<u>Primary prevention:</u> Reducing the likelihood of the unhelpful behaviour by targeting known personal and environmental triggers.

- *Staff may avoid telling off a student in front of the rest of the class if this is a known trigger, instead approaching them in a 1:1 context.*
- *The young person may practice deep breathing before entering a potentially triggering but necessary situation, such as an exam or a detention.*

<u>Secondary Prevention</u>: Reducing the likelihood of the unhelpful behaviour by spotting the early warning signs and reacting before it escalates.

- *If the child has their hood up and is not making eye contact (warning signs) they can be offered a 1:1 chat or a distraction activity (agreed strategies).*
- *If the child recognises their own escalation, they may communicate this to an appropriate adult whilst they are still calm enough to communicate effectively. They may even use the Emotion Thermometer as a communication tool for this.*

<u>Reactive:</u> Responding quickly, effectively, and ethically to the unhelpful behaviour to reduce the severity of its impact and support de-escalation.

- *If the child walks out of the room shouting, they will not be followed OR if they have to be followed for safety reasons staff will not attempt to immediately engage in conversation, instead stating why they are following and leaving appropriate distance.*
- *If the child gets into an argument, they can recognise that they are too high up in their thermometer and choose to exit the room instead of engaging in the argument.*

Activity Information

Facilitators should briefly explain the content of the worksheet. Young people are encouraged to pick one emotion to do the worksheet on (facilitators should encourage young people to focus on the emotion that they are struggling most with). Facilitators may use the 'Emotion Thermometer Prompts' worksheet to support this exercise – some young people may benefit from having these prompts and examples. They may sort the ones provided and add more detail if needed.

Young people should reflect on their thermometer for the chosen emotion and pick a number/ intensity for the following stages:

- After this point I feel 'out of control'.
- After this point I feel uncomfortable or struggling to manage.
- Between these two points I can manage the emotion.

This exercise aims to illustrate how easy or difficult participants find it to cope with their named emotion. These reflections may also help them tailor their adaptive strategies and improve their recognition of when to implement them. Facilitators may wish to prompt a discussion at this point:

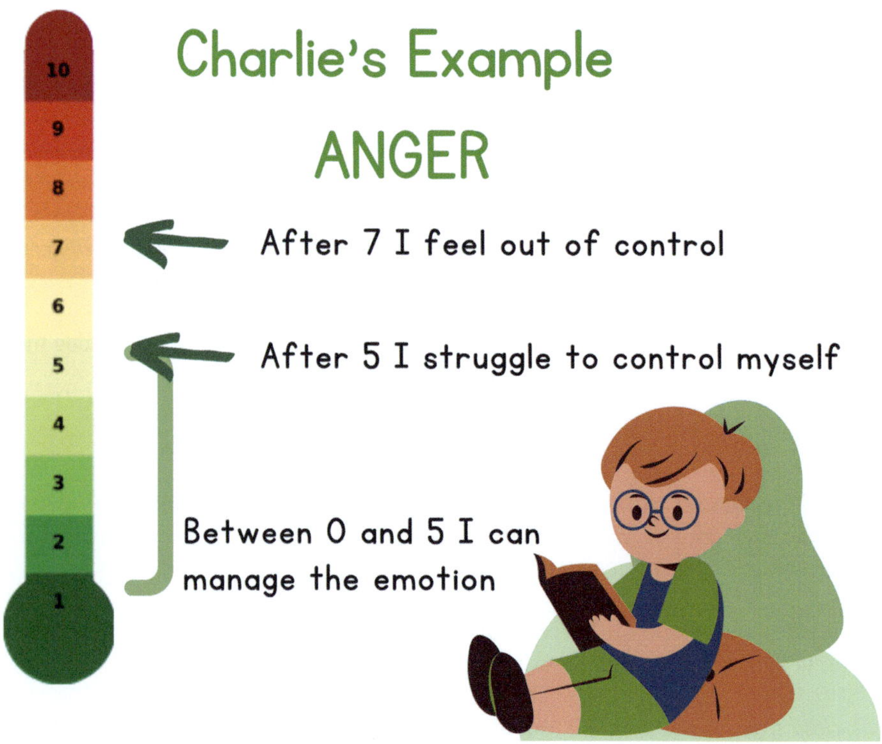

Figure 11.1

- Does everyone start feeling 'out of control' at the same level? What helps some people stay in control at higher intensities?
- Pick a situation that elicits the emotion (e.g. situations that may be frustrating such as someone cutting in line in front of you or shouting at you). Ask the young people to name what number in the thermometer they would feel in that situation. Different people are likely to give different ratings.

This discussion point aims to reassure students that each person is different, and we each have unique needs and tolerances. However, it also helps identify existing strengths in attendees. Facilitators may praise these strengths, motivate attendees, and highlight their abilities to achieve positive change. Identified strengths may also support attendees who are struggling to identify goals and skills to work towards.

After identifying the three main stages of emotion escalation, attendees should add detail to the worksheet by identifying:

- Internal and external warning signs for each stage (e.g. body map/sensations, foot tapping, not making eye contact...)
- Current behaviours at each stage (e.g. walking out, punching a wall...)
  Attendees may benefit from discussing whether their current behaviours fulfil a positive or negative function of the emotion (refer back to session 2's content on the functions of emotions).
- Events that may trigger a quick escalation of the emotion.
  Attendees may benefit from discussing their triggers. They may explore the specifics of what escalates their emotion, adding detail to their understanding.

  Attendees may also support each other by exploring similarities and differences amongst their triggers. Participants may share tips on how they cope with their own triggers OR how they cope with situations which others find triggering. This may identify some useful skills and strategies for other young people to try.

  Attendees should also discuss 'exceptions to the rule' (i.e. times that the trigger has occurred, but they have managed their response). This may help identify protective factors and strategies which they can use to prevent escalation in the future.

After completing the warning signs and behaviours for each stage, attendees can then proceed to naming helpful and unhelpful actions which they can take at each state of escalation.

- Helpful actions are those which help attendees address the problem in a pro-social manner. They may be performed by attendees themselves or by key people in their environment (e.g. staff).
- Unhelpful actions are those which continue to escalate the problem. They may be performed by attendees themselves or by key people in their environment (e.g. staff).

The main goal of discussions within this exercise is to encourage young people to reflect on the similarities and differences in their thermometers. This in turn can help identify strengths within the group, which can allow peers to support each other with strategies. If done respectfully, peers may also challenge each other's perceptions of the behaviours – they may identify if someone has minimised their positives or negatives. For example, they may identify if a peer

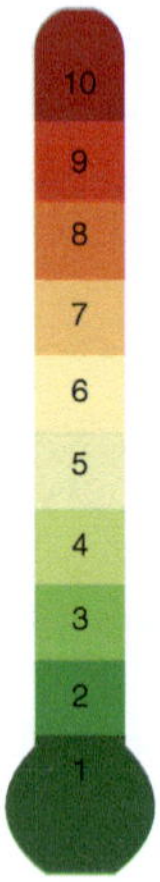

Out of control			
Warning signs	Things i might do	Helpful strategies	Unhelpful things
Struggling to control			
Warning signs	Things i might do	Helpful strategies	Unhelpful things
Managing			
Warning signs	Things i might do	Helpful strategies	Unhelpful things

Figure 11.2

has used a strategy in the past which they have not identified in their work, or if they tend to escalate quicker than they think.

This task also provides the opportunity for facilitators to highlight the link between emotion 'intensity' and the actions of young people. The use of this can be highlighted, for example:

- We may act different at different 'intensity' levels.
- Being aware of what level we are at can inform our choices. Some strategies, such as communicating how we feel, may not be feasible at higher levels of intensity.
- Certain strategies may work better at different levels.
- Using 'back to neutral' strategies can help us calm down.

The completed emotion thermometers should be shared (with the consent of attendees) with key stakeholders in the young person's environment (e.g. school staff, parents) to promote a wide and consistent use of the plan.

Facilitators should take the completed worksheets from attendees (or take pictures of them) to transfer the content into a computer copy, which can be then printed and shared with the young person and relevant others. This will be more structured and readable than a handwritten copy.

Task 3: Introduction to Deep Breathing

Duration: *10 Minutes*
Objectives: *Explore Deep Breathing*
Resources: *Speakers*
Recording or Script
Deep Breathing Leaflet

Facilitators may finish the session with a 'return to neutral' breathing exercise, to continue developing the self-regulation and self-soothing skills[5, 6] of the young people.

Facilitators can demonstrate and guide a short breathing exercise as a final exercise for the session (see 'Deep Breathing' leaflet). Alternatively, facilitators may play a suitable video to guide attendees through deep breathing exercises.

Facilitators should supplement this exercise with the 'Deep Breathing' leaflet, which can be handed out to attendees as a resource to use in their spare time.

Information for Facilitators – Why Do We Practice Deep Breathing?

When we're anxious, angry, or overwhelmed, our breathing becomes fast and shallow, which increases heart rate, muscle tension, and adrenaline. Deep breathing slows the heart rate, lowers blood pressure, and reduces muscle tension, signalling to the body that it is safe.

Shallow breathing can also cause imbalances in oxygen and carbon dioxide levels, which may worsen feelings of panic or dizziness. Deep breathing restores balance, leading to a clearer and calmer state of mind.

Focusing on the breath creates a mindful 'pause' between the emotional trigger and the response. This moment of slowing down can prevent automatic, impulsive reactions and allow for more intentional choices.

Overall, deep breathing is an essential strategy for emotion regulation. It tackles physiological factors, supporting calm and effective functioning of the body and the brain. This, in turn, provides the brain with resources to make better decisions, as opposed to impulsively reacting with the fight or flight instinct.

References

1 Allen, D. (2009). Positive behavioural support as a service system for people with challenging behaviour. *Psychiatry*, *8*(10), 408–412.

2 LaVigna, G.W., & Willis, T.J. (2012). The efficacy of positive behavioural support with the most challenging behaviour: The evidence and its implications. *Journal of Intellectual and Developmental Disability*, *37*(3), 185–195.

3 McClean, B., Grey, I.M., & McCracken, M. (2007). An evaluation of positive behavioural support for people with very severe challenging behaviours in community-based settings. *Journal of Intellectual Disabilities*, *11*(3), 281–301.

4 Allen, D., McGill, P., Hastings, R.P., Toogood, S., Baker, P., Gore, N.J., & Hughes, J.C. (2013). Implementing positive behavioural support: Changing social and organisational contexts. *International Journal of Positive Behavioural Support*, *3*(2), 32–41.

5 Shafir, T. (2015). Movement-based strategies for emotion regulation. In *Handbook on emotion regulation: Processes, cognitive effects and social consequences*, edited by M. L. Bryant (pp. 231–249). Nova Science Publishers.

6 Gillespie, S.M., Mitchell, I.J., Fisher, D., & Beech, A.R. (2012). Treating disturbed emotional regulation in sexual offenders: The potential applications of mindful self-regulation and controlled breathing techniques. *Aggression and Violent Behavior*, *17*(4), 333–343.

12 Session 4

Recognising Emotions in Others

Task 1: Check-In

Duration: 10 Minutes (+ Icebreaker duration)
Objectives: Promote peer support and reflection
Resources: Completed 'Emotion Thermometer' worksheet
This task may be preceded by an icebreaker task.

Facilitators should prompt a review of the content covered the previous week. This may be aided by the completed 'Emotion Thermometer' worksheets. Facilitators should prompt students to reflect on any escalations they have had this week, as well as how young people coped with them:

- What happened?
- What did you do? Was it in line with the plan?
- What did you achieve?
- What would you do differently next time?

Task 2: Emotion Charades and Roleplay

Duration: 30–45 Minutes
Objectives: Promote Engagement
Exploring accuracy when identifying others' emotions
Explore how accuracy may change depending on our emotions and experiences
Promote Empathy and Perspective Taking
Resources: Emotion Wheel which can 'spin' OR papers with 'emotions' in a bag OR software for random selection of prompts
Character Scripts OR Relevant Videos

Part 1: One Emotion at a Time

Facilitators should prepare the resource of choice prior to the session, so that the random allocation of emotions may be easily done during the session.

Young people will take turns, one at a time, at acting out a randomly allocated emotion. The rest of the young people will attempt to guess the emotion.

The way that the exercise is run and rewarded will depend on the group needs. However, one possible way of running it is as follows:

DOI: 10.4324/9781003666738-12

- A 'prize' is presented for the person with the most points to win (smaller prizes may be available for other participants).
- Points are won if your emotion is guessed correctly within 1 minute, and if you guess another person's emotion correctly.
- A spinning wheel can be created using the emotion wheel resource. Participants may earn 1 point if they choose an 'easier' emotion (from the centre) and 2 points if they choose a more 'complex' emotion (from the outside). This allows for participants to take part at a level of complexity which they feel comfortable with whilst still encouraging them to challenge themselves. Emotion charades aim to improve overall literacy and recognition surrounding emotions. This exercise has been successfully used in interventions targeting social and emotional learning,[1] as well as emotion regulation.[2]

Part 2: Emotion Role-Play

Facilitators will provide scripts for the young people which give them emotions and a context for their characters (Sample scripts are provided in the manual). The young people may then interact as their characters for a limited time period. The rest of the young people can observe the interaction. After some role-play, the 'actors' should try to guess each other's emotion. The 'audience' may also have a guess.

**Note: Facilitators may use appropriate videos instead of role-play. This may be beneficial for groups who are reluctant to role-play or for 1:1 delivery.*

If appropriate for the group, rather than guessing the emotion, 'actors' may switch roles. This aims to encourage perspective taking and empathy for others.

At the end of each role-play exercise, facilitators should promote discussion amongst the young people. Some prompts may include:

- Did the actors/audience struggle to identify the emotion? Why/why not?
- How did the emotions affect the way people behaved? Were they helpful? How does this relate to the functions of emotions?
- How did it feel to be Character X? How did it feel when the other character spoke to you?
- How did it feel changing characters? How did it change your approach?
- What would have been a better way for Character X to approach the situation?

The content of Task 2 (Part 2) may continue to be used within Task 3.

This exercise aims to make young people reflect on how they may interpret emotions through the lens of their own emotion. For example, when they are angry, they may be more likely to think that others are angry at them or purposefully annoying them. Another example may be 'rose tinted glasses' – when they are incredibly happy or in love, they may not notice other people being sad or mean. In this way, the tasks improve young people's insight into their own biases when interpreting others' behaviours.[3]

This exercise also aims to improve empathy and perspective taking by encouraging young people to view the situation through another person's eyes.[4] Role play has been widely and successfully used as a method of promoting empathy in a variety of samples, ranging from schoolchildren[5] to offenders.[6, 7] Increased empathy, in turn, results in a reduction of aggressive behaviour and improvements in compassion and conflict resolution.[5, 8]

Maintaining Safety: The character scripts aim to showcase conflict between the characters, as well as possible poor communication. It is important throughout the exercise to maintain awareness of the following:

- Some people may have a history of traumatic experiences and may be affected by the content in these scenarios. It is important during this exercise to monitor the young people and check-in if they seem uncomfortable or upset. Please refer to 'Dealing with difficult issues' for further guidance.
- It may be relevant to give a trigger warning prior to the exercise and encourage young people to speak up if they need a break or become upset (or remind them of the group agreements, if these cover the need for breaks and time-outs).
- It is important to prevent inappropriate use of the role-play exercise. Create clear boundaries prior to the exercise and remind young people of the group agreements (e.g. respect). For example, it may be useful to remind young people that, even though their character/emotion is angry, they cannot insult, hit, or threaten their peers. Facilitators should be acutely aware of peer dynamics when selecting 'actors' for a scenario and should intervene as soon as possible if they observe an 'actor' becoming overly intense in their behaviour. (e.g. shouting, believable threats, invading personal space).
- 'Actors' may be encouraged to sit in a specific chair for their character, as opposed to standing up. This can help facilitators maintain physical distance between actors to prevent invasions of personal space.
- It may also be appropriate to introduce a word or sign which actors can use to stop the roleplay if they need to.

Task 3: Social Stories – A Comic Book Perspective

Duration: *20 Minutes*
Objectives: *Explore how accuracy may change depending on our emotions and experiences*
Promote Empathy and Perspective Taking
Resources: *'Social Story' Worksheet*

Facilitators may use the following sources to prompt young people with content for the social story worksheet:

- Content of Task 2 – the character scripts and/or discussions had by the 'actors' in character.
- Suggestions from staff at the host organisation (e.g. school teachers) – they may provide realistic scenarios which they have observed and are relevant to the young people.
- Suggestions from the young people – they may provide examples of observed or lived conflict scenarios.

This task should be led by a collaborative discussion. A scenario may be suggested to tackle as a group. The 'social story' may be adapted to include the number of characters featuring in the scenario.

For each character, the social story/ comic strip encourages young people to consider:

- What is the person saying? What is their voice tone?
- What do they look like? (Facial expression, posture)

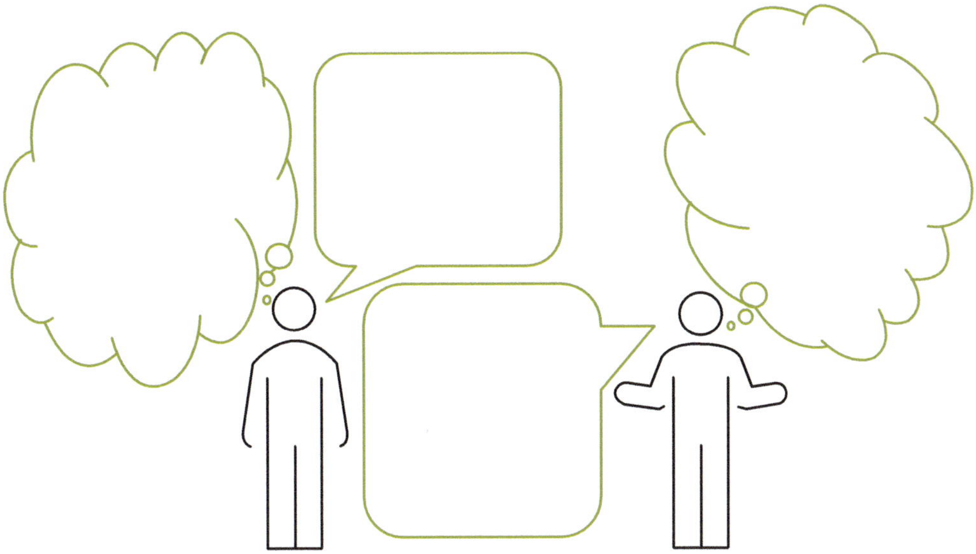

Figure 12.1

- What is the person thinking? Consider how their history and emotions may affect their thoughts. For example, a history of bullying may mean the person feels insecure and thinks that everyone hates them (Refer back to the ecological model in session 1)
- How is the person feeling?

Example:

Sam and Jessie are friends who are hanging out together.

Sam's perspective: Sam is waiting for results to a test they had at the doctors. They don't want to tell Jessie about this, as they feel embarrassed about the problem. If they miss the phone call from the doctor, they've been told they won't be able to speak to the doctor for another week. Sam keeps looking at their phone to make sure they don't miss the call. Sam is struggling to listen to what Jessie is saying.

Jessie's perspective: Jessie has recently broken up with a partner and was looking forward to meeting up with Sam to talk to a friend about it. Sam keeps looking at their phone and doesn't seem to be listening. Jessie continues to try to talk to Sam but gets more and more wound up as this goes on.

Social stories are an intervention widely used with individuals with Autism Spectrum Disorders (ASD).[9] Although the underlying mechanisms driving the effects of this intervention remain speculative.[10] social stories have been linked to moderate improvements in perspective taking and emotion recognition.[9, 11] Social stories have also shown effectiveness at reducing inappropriate or disruptive behaviours amongst children with learning disabilities (LD).[12] Research has also suggested feasibility in adapting the use of social stories to a larger sample of young people with behavioural difficulties, beyond those with ASD diagnoses.[13]

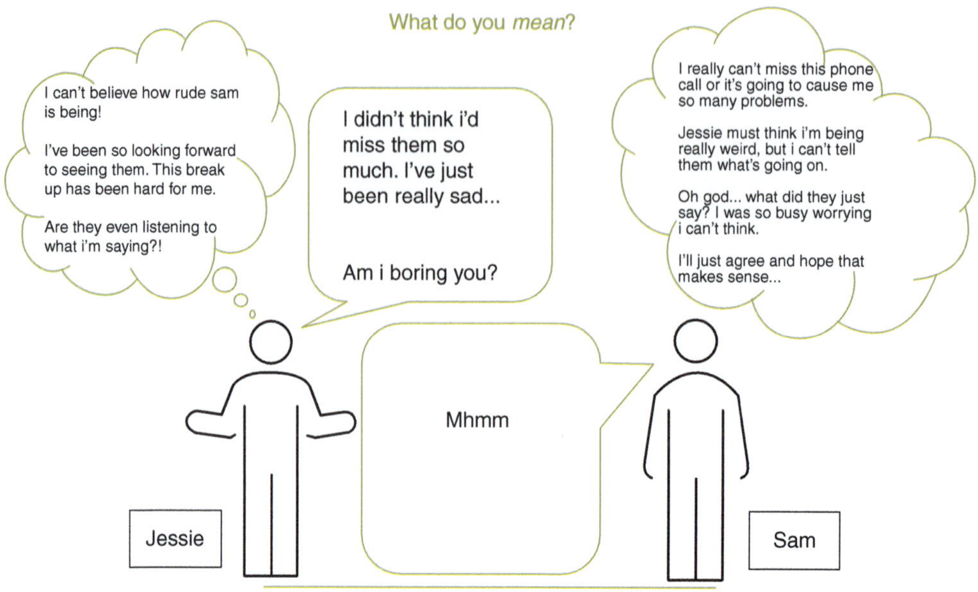

Figure 12.2

Task 4: Introduction to Mindfulness and Relaxation

Duration: *5 Minutes*
Objectives: *Explore Mindfulness*
Resources: *Speakers*
Recording, App or Script

Facilitators may finish the session with a 'return to neutral' (e.g. mindfulness, relaxation) exercise, to continue developing the self-regulation and self-soothing skills[14] of the young people.

In this session, it may be beneficial to introduce an easily accessible resource which young people can use at home between sessions. Examples of this may include:

- Free to use Apps: Breathe2Relax, Headspace (free trial)
- Relevant YouTube videos
- Relevant websites. For example, ChildLine has a free-to-access resource where children and young people can build their own 'safe place' ('Build your happy place' on childline.org.uk)
- Calming Phone Apps: This is sand, Pause, Gravitarium
- Any other relevant resources you can think of!

Facilitators can demonstrate and guide the use of these as a final exercise to the session. It may be useful to supplement this with a resource sheet which young people can take home to search the resources.

References

1 Tan, K., Wegmann, K., Patino, R., Hand, B., Mitchell, J., & Moser, K. (2021). Social and Emotional Learning Group Work during the COVID-19 pandemic, the reopening, and the mobilization for racial justice. *Children & Schools*, *43*(2), 118–122.

2 Southam-Gerow, M.A. (2013). *Emotion regulation in children and adolescents: A practitioner's guide*. Guilford Press.

3 Prutzman, P., & Johnson, J. (1997). Bias awareness and multiple perspectives: Essential aspects of conflict resolution. *Theory into Practice*, *36*(1), 26–31.

4 Weisz, E., & Zaki, J. (2017). Empathy building interventions: A review of existing work and suggestions for future directions. In *The Oxford handbook of compassion science*, edited by E. M. Seppälä, E. Simon Thomas, S. L. Brown, M. C. Worline, L. Cameron and J. R. Doty (pp. 205–217). Oxford University Press.

5 Castillo, R., Salguero, J.M., Fernández-Berrocal, P., & Balluerka, N. (2013). Effects of an emotional intelligence intervention on aggression and empathy among adolescents. *Journal of Adolescence*, *36*(5), 883–892.

6 Pithers, W.D. (1999). Empathy: Definition, enhancement, and relevance to the treatment of sexual abusers. *Journal of Interpersonal Violence*, *14*(3), 257–284.

7 Webster, S.D., Bowers, L.E., Mann, R.E., & Marshall, W.L. (2005). Developing empathy in sexual offenders: The value of offence re-enactments. *Sexual Abuse: A Journal of Research and Treatment*, *17*(1), 63–77.

8 Klimecki, O.M. (2019). The role of empathy and compassion in conflict resolution. *Emotion Review*, *11*(4), 310–325.

9 Bellini, S., & Peters, J.K. (2008). Social skills training for youth with autism spectrum disorders. *Child and Adolescent Psychiatric Clinics of North America*, *17*(4), 857–873.

10 Reynhout, G., & Carter, M. (2011). Social stories™: A possible theoretical rationale. *European Journal of Special Needs Education*, *26*(3), 367–378.

11 Otero, T.L., Schatz, R.B., Merrill, A.C., & Bellini, S. (2015). Social skills training for youth with autism spectrum disorders: A follow-up. *Child and Adolescent Psychiatric Clinics*, *24*(1), 99–115.

12 Kalyva, E., & Agaliotis, I. (2009). Can social stories enhance the interpersonal conflict resolution skills of children with LD? *Research in Developmental Disabilities*, *30*(1), 192–202.

13 Whitehead, J. (2007). Telling it like it is: Developing social stories™ for children in mainstream primary schools. *Pastoral Care in Education*, *25*(4), 35–41.

14 Leyland, A., Rowse, G., & Emerson, L. M. (2019). Experimental effects of mindfulness inductions on self-regulation: Systematic review and meta-analysis. *Emotion*, *19*(1), 108.

13 Session 5

Mental Mistakes

Task 1: Check-In

Duration: 10 Minutes (+ Icebreaker duration)
Objectives: Promote peer support and reflection
Resources: None

Facilitators should regularly check in with attendees regarding their attitudes and applications of the work covered. Session 5 marks the mid-point for SHERBET and may thus be an ideal time to review progress, as it may inform adjustments in delivery. Some useful prompts may include:

- How are you finding the sessions so far?
- Are they what you expected? Why/why not?
- What are some things that you have found useful in SHERBET so far?
- How are you getting on with your goal?
- Have you used anything that you learned in sessions outside of sessions (e.g. at school, at home...)? How did it go?

It may be particularly useful to check the development of insight and empathy in the young people, following Session 3. For example:

- Last week we looked at challenging disagreements and miscommunications. Have you encountered anything like them this week? What happened? What did you do?
- Have you used any 'return to neutral' strategies? When/why? Did they help?
- Is it easy/hard to think of arguments from the other person's perspective? Do you try to do it? How did you find it last week? Have you used this skill since our last session?

The prompts above may all hold some relevance but it is not necessary to cover all of them. Facilitators can promote collaborative working by expanding on the prompts which young people respond to the most.

Check-ins can be used to gain an understanding of the young people, as well as build rapport. In particular, understanding the attitudes, engagement and interest of the young people can help us assess their progress and tailor their support.

DOI: 10.4324/9781003666738-13

Task 2: Session 3 Review – Communication Flow

Duration: *25 Minutes*
Objectives: *Promote peer support and reflection*
Promote empathy and perspective taking
Promote competent communication
Resources: *Social stories or character scripts used last session*
If working with a quick group, some new scenarios for discussion

This exercise builds on the content of the previous session. Reflecting on the scenarios covered, young people should be encouraged to identify what elements may 'break' the flow of communication, and what the impact of this may be. This may be assisted with a 'social stories' worksheet for visual reference.

What Is Communication? – Information for Facilitators

Communication encompasses all the transmitting and receiving of information, regardless of format (e.g. phone call, text message, talking, letters, signs...). Communication is so important for humans that back in 300 BC, famous philosopher Aristotle was already thinking and teaching how one could become a better communicator[1]. Communication helps us understand the world and be understood by others; it can help us express what we need and negotiate ways of getting it.

However, communication is not always easy and there are many 'moving parts' which can have an impact on the quality of our communication. This manual explains the different elements of communication using a simplified version of Berlo's SMCR model[2]. A simplified version has been used to be more easily understood and utilised by staff and attendees, whilst still explaining the key elements which impact the quality of our communication.

Please note that this model may be further simplified by facilitators if so needed, to improve accessibility.

Berlo's SMCR Model – Adapted

The Context: Where is the communication happening?

- Are any other people present? Who are they?
- Is the context formal (e.g. school) or informal (e.g. a party)?
- Is the context calm/busy/loud...?

The Sender (and encoding): This person creates and sends the message. They create the idea in their heads of what they want to communicate, and they create a message out of this idea (encoding). Things that may affect the sender include:

- Communication Skills: How good are they at listening, writing, speaking...?
- Mood/Attitude: How are they feeling? What are their thoughts and feelings?
- Knowledge: How much does the person know about the subject they're talking about?

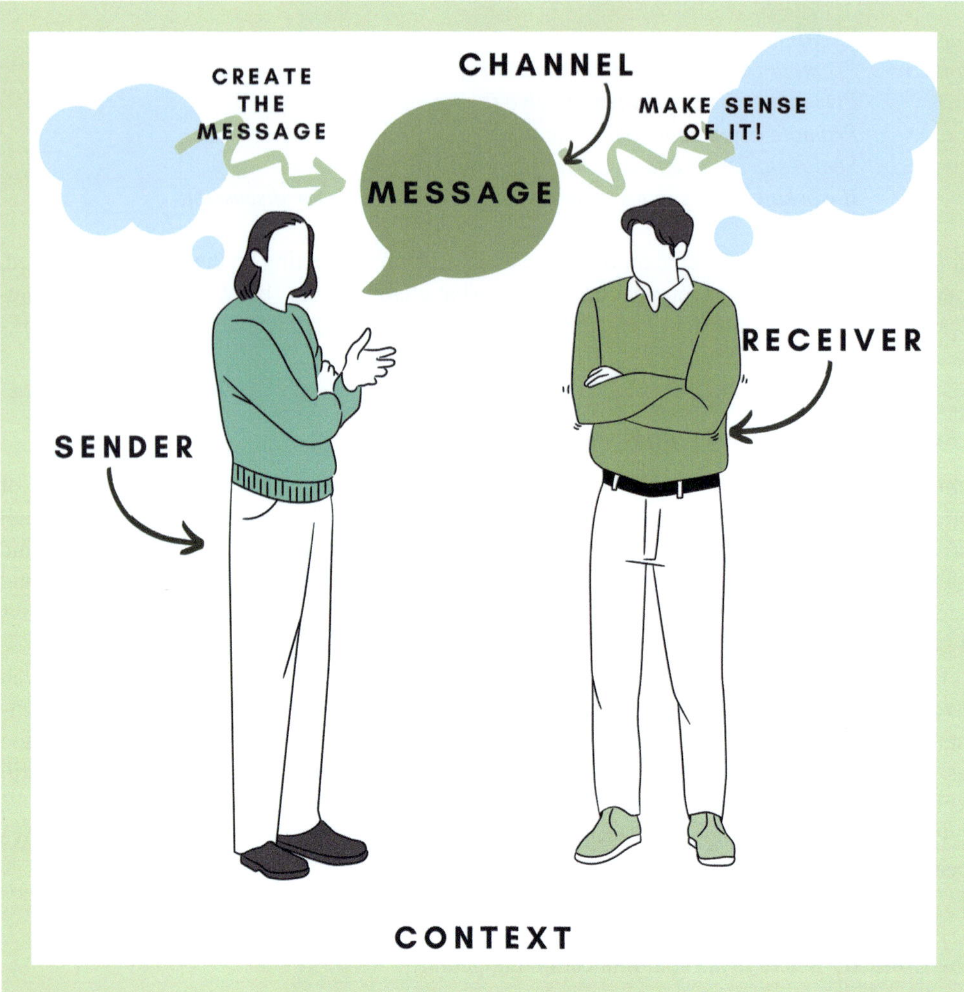

Figure 13.1

- Culture, Personal Experiences, Values: Think back to the work we did on 'The world around us' (Session 1). We explored how social media, family, country and more can affect our lives, our thoughts and our actions. That is still relevant when we communicate!

The Message: This is the information sent from sender to receiver. The sender always has a plan or idea of how the message should be interpreted. In most cases the receiver will find it easy to understand the message accurately.

- Content: What exactly does the message say?
- Non-verbal content: What other elements are affecting the message? Do they change its meaning? For example, tone of voice, gestures, facial expressions.

- Code: Is there a specific content to the message that may not be understood by everyone? For example, emoji, slang, technical language...

The Channel: How the message is sent. This may include by talking in person, by phone call, text message, letter and many more. Are there any limitations to the channel? For example, trying to talk at a noisy party.

The Receiver (and decoding): This is the person who receives the message. They will be affected by the same factors as the sender, and this may impact how they interpret the message and how they react to it!

What Affects Communication?

Facilitators may support young people by highlighting any relevant factors which were not identified in the initial discussion. Some factors impacting the effectiveness of communication include:

- Personal History
  We are designed to learn from what we see and experience[3]. This may make us more aware of certain dangers, more likely to feel judged, or simply change how we communicate.
  - A young person who has been bullied for a long time (maybe at school, maybe at home) may be wary of people showing them kindness and think they are trying to trick them. After all, they have learned that other people are unkind and cannot be trusted!
  - A young person who has grown up in a house where their carers regularly argue and shout at each other may believe this is normal and appropriate for resolving conflict. They may not know other ways to communicate when upset or angry.
- Society and Family Influences:
  Remember the ecological model[4] ('The world around us')? We learned that our relationships, communities and societies can affect our lives. How might this impact our communication?
  - Someone may be more 'defensive' and aggressive if they are in front of their friends, because they are worried of being made fun of if they don't act like their friends expect.
  - Some families or communities may have strict expectations regarding how people should behave – how may this affect a young person?
  - Thinking more widely: How might a person's gender, ethnicity, cultural background... affect how they react and communicate in certain situations? For example, a young Black male may be more afraid or defensive when encountering police because of historical discrimination and criminalisation of ethnic minorities.[5, 6]
- Communication Channel[7]
  Are you communicating in person, over the phone, through text...?
  - How does this impact your ability to understand a person's tone? How do you know if they're joking or being sarcastic?
  - How does your communication change over the phone/over text? Are you more likely to be mean because you cannot see their face? Or are you more likely to think before you respond because you have that time and distance?
- Non-Verbal Communication[9, 10]
  This may include facial expressions, gestures, eye contact, posture, space, tone of voice... How may these affect the communication?

  - For example, a young person may stay quiet in an argument. However, they may still present as intimidating due to their facial expression, posture... This may lead to an escalation of the argument.

  Please note that, although non-verbal communication is a lot more automatic and harder to control than verbal communication – we can still practice our skills and challenge it. Even if the first instinct is to make an angry facial expression, being aware of our non-verbal communication is the first step to modifying it.
- Verbal Communication

  The words we use are also important! Consider the impact of:
  - Insults or disrespectful language
  - Hyper specific language (e.g. technical language, slang...)
  - Coherence – are you expressing yourself in a way others can follow? Does it make sense?
  - Pace – what speed are you talking at?
- Emotion

  As explored in previous sessions, emotions may impact our behaviour and choices.[11] If we are too high in our emotion thermometer we may not be able to use our communication skills effectively. This also applies to the listener – if they are too 'intense' in an emotion, they may not be able to hear what we have to say or communicate well either.
- Bias

  Cognitive biases[12] can impact how we communicate. These likely relate to our personal history (For example, if you have been bullied you may believe that others are generally unkind so you can't trust them.). We will explore this further in Task 3.
- And Many More
  - Language barriers – English may not be their first language.
  - Other special needs, Autism Spectrum Disorder, Learning Disabilities...

It is essential for facilitators to highlight that none of these are excuses for our behaviours. They are explanations for why communication may break down. By being aware of the signs, we can recognise them in ourselves and change them so we may improve how we communicate.

Young people may be involved in the discussion of the model by being prompted to identify **how** changes to the elements may affect communication. Examples may include:

- Being told off in front of your friends/by yourself (context change)
- Being asked a favour by your best friend/by a stranger (sender change)
- Being asked to 'please lower your voice'/'shut up' by someone (message change)
- Sending a sarcastic joke over text/saying it in person (channel change)
- A friend making a joke about your shoes on a day you are feeling happy/on a bad day when you are already annoyed (receiver)

Young people may also contribute their own relevant examples of miscommunication. Facilitators should then prompt young people to think back to the 'circles of control' they covered in Session 1. If the young person was the 'sender' what elements would be in their circle of control/influence/concern?[13] Why?

This may help facilitators identify the strengths and weaknesses of each attendee's communication skills (e.g. how confident are they in crafting a good message? Do they realise their influence over context?).

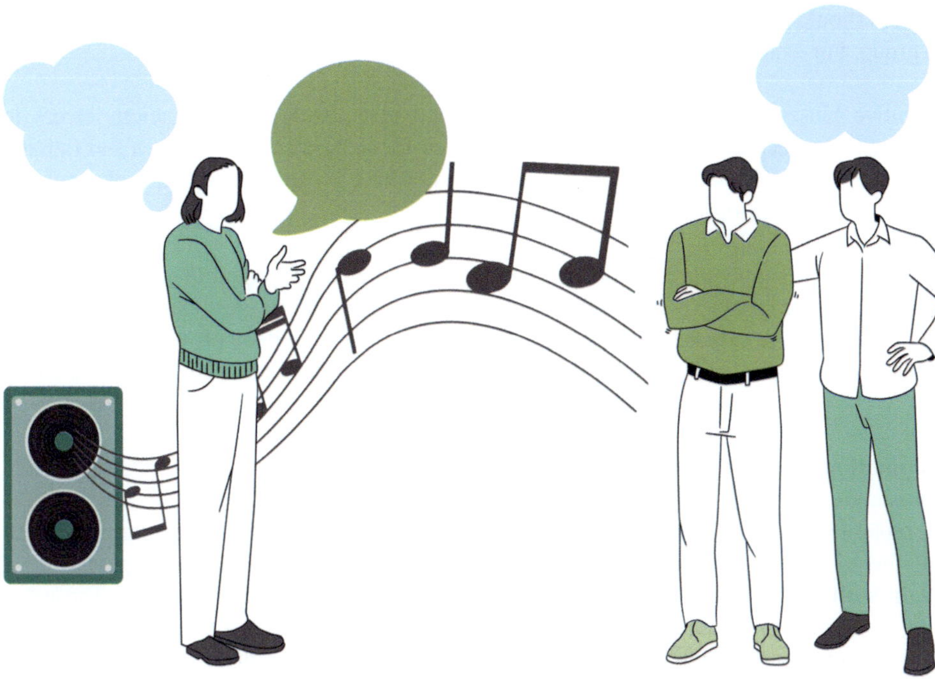

Figure 13.2

Example Situation for Discussion

Mark and Charlie are at a party. Mark seems to be in a bad mood and is ignoring Charlie. Mark's older brother is at the party too and is hanging out nearby.

Charlie is worried about his friend and wants to see if he can help. He asks Mark 'What is wrong with you?'

Mark does not answer. Charlie thinks he can't hear him over the music, so he taps Mark's shoulder and says louder 'Hey, what's wrong with you?'

Mark gets very angry and shoves Charlie saying, 'What's your bloody problem?!'

<u>Mark's perspective:</u>

Mark's older brother teases him a lot and makes fun of him. One common comment is how Mark is not 'man enough' and gets pushed around.

Mark is frustrated and distracted.

When Charlie taps his shoulder and is shouting, Mark interprets the message as Charlie trying to pick a fight. Mark does not want to be embarrassed in front of his brother. He gets surprised and annoyed and reacts by pushing Charlie away.

Task 3: Cognitive Bias

Duration: *30 Minutes*
Objectives: *Promote competent communication*
Teach about cognitive bias
Promote insight and reflection about young people's own biases
Resources: *'Cognitive biases' worksheet*

Facilitators may expand upon the previous exercise by highlighting the role of cognitive biases.[14] Facilitators should provide a definition for cognitive biases adapted to the communication needs of the group. For example:

> Cognitive biases (a.k.a. 'thinking errors', 'mental mistakes') are unconscious errors in thinking that affect how we see the word around us, meaning that we see it in a less rational or accurate way. These are automatic processes, which we developed to make quicker decisions. However, they can also be unhelpful.

Facilitators and young people may then collaboratively explore some common cognitive biases, supported by the 'cognitive biases' worksheet. Young people may suggest examples for when they have observed or experienced each cognitive bias. Some have been provided here in case young people struggle to identify examples. The cognitive biases covered in the worksheet include:

- **Rumination or 'Sticky Thoughts'** – This is a state where we may get 'stuck' in a specific thought. Overthinking can lead to the emotion getting more intense.
  Example: Lying in bed late at night thinking about a time when you felt embarrassed. You only feel more embarrassed and uncomfortable, and it's stopping you from sleeping.
- **All or Nothing Thinking** – As the name says, this describes extremes in thinking. These can refer to yourself or to other people. Some 'all or nothing' expressions you may have heard are: 'If I'm not perfect, I have failed', 'Either I do it right or not at all'.
  Example: I really tried to study for this test and only got an 8/10. It's not a 10/10, so I am really disappointed and embarrassed. I think there is no point in even trying next time.
- **Over Generalising** – Seeing a pattern in a single event, making generalised conclusions. Some common words associated with this are: Never, always, nothing, everything... For example, 'everything is always rubbish'.
  Example: I got a bad grade on a test, so I must be horrible at school.
- **Mental Filter** – Paying attention to certain evidence.
  Example: When I am angry with my family I can only think of all the times they have upset me. I don't pay attention to the times they have done nice things or all the things they do for me.
- **Disqualifying the Positive** – Saying that when something positive happens 'it doesn't count'.
  Example: You get a good grade in a test and think it must have just been lucky because you are not good at school.
- **Magnification** – Blowing things out of proportion.
  Example: My best friend and I argued. If I don't have her, I literally have no one to talk to, so what is the point in life. I will never make friends again.
- **Minimisation** – 'Shrinking' something to make it seem less important.
  Example: I got into a fight and hurt someone. But I pretend, maybe even believe, that it's not a big deal. They didn't even get that hurt. They should have seen it coming. It's not even my fault.
- **Critical Words** – Using critical words like 'should', 'must' or 'ought' can make us feel guilty, or like we have already failed. This is also true when we say them to other people – they will likely feel frustrated.
  Example: (When recovering from a mental health or physical health problem, a lot of people experience this thought): I should be better by now.

- **Emotional Reasoning** – Assuming that because we feel a certain way, what we think must be true.
  Example: I am really upset and sad, so my life must be horrible.
- **Jumping to Conclusions** – Can include 'mind reading' (imagining that we know what others are thinking) or 'fortune telling' (imagining that we know what is going to happen).
  Example: My parents grounded me so I cannot see my friends. I think they did it on purpose to annoy me, they just want me to miss out.

Throughout this exercise it is important for facilitators to promote a compassionate, yet change-oriented, approach. Cognitive biases tend to develop out of need and function. For example:

- Research highlights the evolutionary advantages of cognitive biases, which at points may have been adaptive[14] (e.g. beliefs about danger, the co-cooperativeness of others...).
- Cognitive biases may also arise as the consequence of traumatic events (e.g. people who experienced acute stress disorder following a motor-vehicle accident were more likely to exhibit biases, exaggerating the probability of negative events happening).[15]

Facilitators should be aware that some young people may have experienced life events which contributed to the development of unhelpful biases and behaviours. However, it is worth highlighting to the young people that, although those adaptations made sense at the time (e.g. cavemen were hypervigilant of danger to keep the tribe safe), they are unhelpful now (e.g. hypervigilance in the modern world may lead to aggression and anxiety). This allows facilitators to encourage young people to change and develop better strategies, whilst still showing empathy and compassion for the circumstances in which unhelpful biases were developed.

It may also be worth highlighting that cognitive biases act in our thoughts, not our behaviours. Therefore, by being aware of the existence of cognitive biases, we can recognise them and try to 'think differently'. Even if we cannot 'think differently' straight away, recognising that a thought may be inaccurate or unhelpful can help us ignore it when making choices and 'act differently' (e.g. some people may have grown up in a racist environment but they can recognise when they have a racist thought and challenge it or dismiss it, so it doesn't affect their behaviour).

Overall, thinking biases show us that we may not be responsible for the first thought that pops into our mind. However, we are responsible for the second thought, and responsible for the resulting action.

Task 4: Thought-Based Mindfulness and Relaxation

Duration: 5 Minutes
Objectives: Explore mindfulness
Resources: Script, included below

Facilitators may finish the session with a 'return to neutral' (e.g. mindfulness, relaxation) exercise, to continue developing the self-regulation and self-soothing skills[16] of the young people. A thought-based mindfulness exercise is recommended, as it links to the content of the session (i.e. cognitive biases).

A thought-based mindfulness exercise is a practice where the focus of attention is on your thoughts themselves, rather than the breath, body or external environment. Instead of trying to change or stop thoughts, you practice noticing them with curiosity and without judgment. This helps you build awareness of your mental patterns and reduces the tendency to get 'hooked' by unhelpful thoughts.[17]

Mindfulness Exercise: Clouds in the Sky

Take a comfortable seat. Let your hands rest gently, and if you feel comfortable, close your eyes.

Begin by taking a slow, deep breath in… and a gentle, long breath out.

Now, imagine a wide, open sky above you. It's clear, spacious, endless. This sky represents your mind – a big space where your attention and thoughts live.

As you sit here, thoughts may begin to appear. Imagine each thought as a cloud drifting across the sky.

Some clouds may be small and wispy – like quick, passing thoughts. Others may be heavier or darker – like worries, judgments or memories.

Whatever the cloud looks like, simply notice it. You don't need to chase it, push it away, or hold onto it. Just watch it drift across the open sky of your mind.

If you notice yourself getting caught up in a cloud – maybe following a story, or analysing it – that's okay. The moment you notice, gently bring your awareness back to the sky itself, and allow the thought-cloud to keep moving.

There's no need to control the sky. Just notice: thoughts start, thoughts pass. Clouds come, clouds go.

Take a few breaths as you watch the flow of clouds – observing with kindness, patience and curiosity.

And when you're ready, gently bring your attention back to your body. Feel the support of the ground beneath you. Take a final deep breath in… and a long breath out.

When you're ready, open your eyes.

References

1 Van Noorden, S. (1993). A translation of Aristotle's Rhetoric-George A. Kennedy: Aristotle, on Rhetoric: A theory of civic discourse. Pp. 335. New York and Oxford: Oxford University Press, 1991. $27.95. *The Classical Review*, *43*(2), 251–252.

2 Stead, B. A. (1972). Berlo's communication process model as applied to the behavioral theories of Maslow, Herzberg, and McGregor. *Academy of Management Journal*, *15*(3), 389–394.

3 Bandura, A., & Walters, R. H. (1977). *Social learning theory* (Vol. 1). Englewood cliffs.

4 Bronfenbrenner, U. (1992). *Ecological systems theory*. Jessica Kingsley Publishers.

5 Yesufu, S. (2013). Discriminatory use of police stop-and-search powers in London, UK. *International Journal of Police Science & Management*, *15*(4), 281–293.

6 Souhami, A. (2014). Institutional racism and police reform: An empirical critique. *Policing and Society*, *24*(1), 1–21.

7 Scissors, L., & Gergle, D. (2016). On the bias: Self-esteem biases across communication channels during romantic couple conflict. In *Proceedings of the 19th ACM Conference on Computer-Supported Cooperative Work & Social Computing* (pp. 383–393).

8 Westmyer, S. A., DiCioccio, R. L., & Rubin, R. B. (1998). Appropriateness and effectiveness of communication channels in competent interpersonal communication. *Journal of Communication*, *48*(3), 27–48.

9 Hinde, R. A., & Hinde, R. A. (Eds.). (1972). *Non-verbal communication*. Cambridge University Press.

10 Burgoon, J. K., Manusov, V., & Guerrero, L. K. (2021). *Nonverbal communication*. Routledge.

11 Kanske, P. (2012). On the influence of emotion on conflict processing. *Frontiers in Integrative Neuroscience*, *6*, 42.

12 Haselton, M. G., Nettle, D., & Murray, D. R. (2015). The evolution of cognitive bias. In *The handbook of evolutionary psychology*, edited by D. M. Buss (pp. 1–20). Wiley.

13 Covey, S. R. (2004). *The 7 habits of highly effective people: Powerful lessons in personal change*. Simon and Schuster.

14 Haselton, M. G., Nettle, D., & Murray, D. R. (2015). The evolution of cognitive bias. In *The handbook of evolutionary psychology*, edited by D. M. Bus (pp. 1–20). Wiley.

15 Warda, G., & Bryant, R. A. (1998). Cognitive bias in acute stress disorder. *Behaviour Research and Therapy*, *36*(12), 1177–1183.

16 Leyland, A., Rowse, G., & Emerson, L. M. (2019). Experimental effects of mindfulness inductions on self-regulation: Systematic review and meta-analysis. *Emotion*, *19*(1), 108.

17 Hayes, S. C., Strosahl, K. D., & Wilson, K. G. (2012). *Acceptance and commitment therapy: The process and practice of mindful change* (2nd ed.). The Guilford Press.

14 Session 6

Thoughts, Feelings and Behaviours

Task 1: Check-In

Duration: *10 Minutes (+ Icebreaker duration)*
Objectives: *Promote peer support and reflection*
Resources: *None*

Facilitators can prompt the attendees to reflect on the content from the previous week to check participants' understanding and application of this knowledge.

This may be done by asking young people about their week: Have they encountered any situations where they have used what they have learned in sessions? For example, reflecting on the other person's point of view when having a disagreement or realising that they were stuck on a thinking error.

It may also be useful to test attendees' recall by asking the group to see how many types of thinking errors they can remember without looking at their notes.

Session 5 brings together the content from previous sessions, explicitly showing the link between thoughts, feelings, behaviours and sensations (CBT Model; Beck & Beck, 2011[1]). Having the chance to review and refresh the content at the beginning of the session may make it easier for attendees to engage and understand the rest of the session.

Task 2: The CBT Model (or *The Hot Cross Bun*)

Duration: *45 Minutes*
Objectives: *Teach about the links between thoughts, feelings, behaviours and sensations*
Relate to the information learned so far (e.g. feelings in the body, thought biases, strategies...)
Promote awareness of own CBT cycles
Resources: *CBT model worksheet*
Whiteboard or flipchart for example CBT model

Thoughts, feelings, behaviours and physical sensations are the key factors through which we experience the world and interpret situations around us. Both facilitators and attendees should have some understanding about all these elements, as sessions 1–4 covered:

- How emotions feel; including valence, intensity and how they feel in the body.
- The functions of emotions and how they affect our behaviours.
- Thought biases and how they affect our interactions.

DOI: 10.4324/9781003666738-14

The influence which these factors have on each other would have been observed by attendees in previous sessions. However, this exercise allows for the explicit exploration of these relationships.

Brief Explanation of CBT – For Facilitators

Cognitive Behavioural Therapy (CBT; Beck & Beck, 2011[1]) is a therapeutic model which focuses on the present moment. Instead of exploring a client's past, CBT focuses on identifying the current difficulties and building skills so that clients can manage them now and in the future.

CBT uses a 'hot cross bun' model to help break down the presenting problems into detailed chunks. This helps clients better understand their problems and how they are maintained. It also allows clients to identify where to start introducing strategies to manage the problems.

CBT explains that thoughts, feelings, behaviours and physical sensations allow us to interpret the world and situations which we find ourselves in. For example:

When we encounter ourselves in a stressful situation (e.g. exam is about to start) we may feel nervous (feeling), our heart may speed up (sensation), we may start thinking about how important it is to do well in the exam (thoughts) and we may then start revising in our head some things that we studied (behaviour).

CBT poses that thoughts, feelings, behaviours and sensations are all inter-connected and can influence each other. When individuals fall into unhelpful 'cycles' these internal mechanisms may react in unhelpful or distressing ways. For example:

Mary is in a very important exam (situation). She has prepared well but is a little nervous (feeling). She starts worrying that she has not studied enough, and gets thoughts that she is going to fail, and this will ruin her plans for university (thoughts). Mary's heart starts pounding and her hands are shaking (sensations). She feels anxious and terrified of starting the exam (feelings). Mary is so worked up that she cannot concentrate (sensations) which makes her even more stressed (feelings). Mary leaves the exam room crying (behaviour) because she 'can't do this'.

However, there is still hope for Mary! This model helps individuals identify how their own thoughts and behaviours impact their emotions. Firstly, this helps build an understanding of how the problem maintains itself (e.g. Mary's thoughts add to her stress, and running out of the room only makes the fear of failing worse!).

Secondly, CBT explains that, because all four factors impact each other, making changes in the cycle of influence can help us break it. CBT acknowledges that it is near impossible to change feelings and sensations directly (e.g. telling someone to be 'less anxious' is unlikely to be a successful approach!). However, changes in our thoughts and our actions can help us tackle our problems and manage our feelings, so that we can achieve our goals. For example:

Mary is in a very important exam (situation). She is stressed (feeling) and starts worrying that she is going to fail (thoughts), this makes her heart speed up (sensation). However, Mary takes some deep breaths (behaviour) and thinks about how hard she has studied, repeating to herself in her head that she has done the best she can and she had scored well in her mock exams (thoughts). Mary now feels a bit calmer (feeling) which allows her to focus (sensation) and she starts writing the exam.

Overall CBT helps clients focus on the present problem, breaks it into manageable chunks so that individuals may better understand it. With that understanding clients can then practice

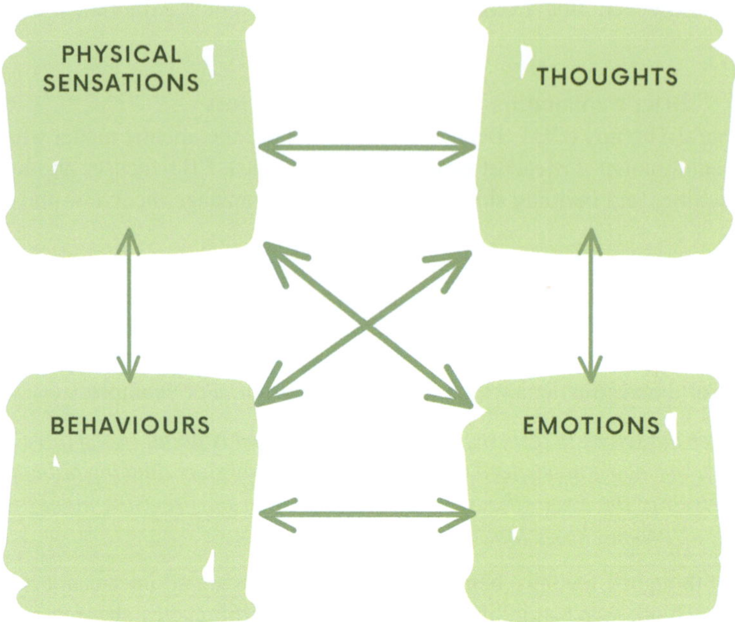

Figure 14.1

improving their thoughts and behaviours so that they can overcome their barriers and achieve their goals. This model has been highly effective in treating symptoms and reducing remission of both internalising (e.g. anxiety, depression, Obsessive Compulsive Disorder, Post-Traumatic Stress Disorder; Riise et al., 2021[2]) and externalising disorders (e.g. ADHD, Conduct Disorder, Oppositional Defiant Disorder; Wergeland et al., 2021[3]) amongst children and adolescents.

Facilitators should introduce a blank CBT cycle or 'hot cross bun'. They should explain that thoughts, feelings, behaviours and sensations shape the way that we experience the world. Young people may then assist by calling out examples of thoughts, feelings, behaviours and sensations to fill in the 'bubbles' in the diagram.

At this point it is essential that facilitators **watch out for confusions between thoughts and feelings.** For example, 'feeling like nothing matters' would not be placed within a CBT model – instead it would be broken down into the thought ('nothing matters') and the feeling ('disappointed, hurt, sad...'). This is a common difficulty encountered when starting to use a CBT approach, as these expressions are commonly used. However, in order to promote appropriate reflections, it is important that facilitators recognise and correct these confusions.

When presenting the CBT cycle to attendees, facilitators may benefit from introducing the concept of 'hot' and 'cold' strategies.

Through these concepts, facilitators and attendees can explore the usefulness of thoughts, behaviours and strategies by considering their consequences in relation to the problem.

Figure 14.2

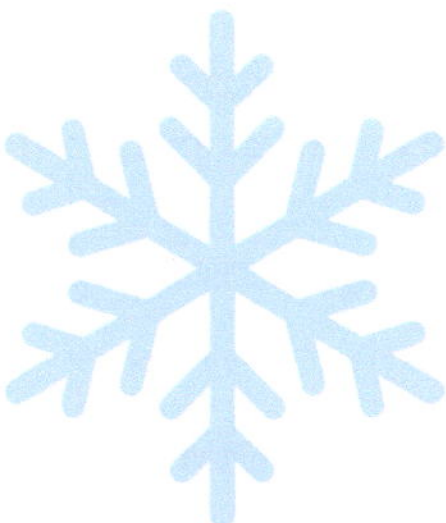

Figure 14.3

Activity 1 – Becoming a Detective

Once the young people have become comfortable with the concepts of thoughts, feelings, behaviours and sensations, facilitators should highlight that they are all linked and they can influence each other (e.g. looking at the arrows in the diagram).

Facilitators should encourage attendees to take a 'detective' approach. This will involve trying to figure out how these connections work and giving examples:

- Emotions and sensations
  - We have explored that we 'feel emotions in the body' (e.g. clenching fists when angry)
  - OR we may experience sensations that affect our emotions (e.g. fast heart rate may make us feel anxious)
- Emotions and thoughts
  - Feeling negative or positive may change how we interpret situations (e.g. when you are scared, thinking that others are out to get you)
  - Our thoughts may change how we feel (e.g. if we think someone is laughing at us we may get angry)

- Emotions and behaviours
  - When you feel scared, you may behave in ways that make you feel safer (e.g. avoiding places that scare you or make you feel anxious)
  - Our actions can change our mood (e.g. doing something you like may make you happy)
- Thoughts and behaviours
  - What we think about a situation may affect how we react to it. (e.g. we are more likely to do things that we like or that matter to us)
  - How we behave can change how we think (e.g. we may think something is scary but once we do it we realise it's not that bad)
- Thoughts and sensations
  - What we think may cause our body to react (e.g. if I think that I am in danger my body may start preparing to fight or flight)
  - We may interpret body sensations in a way that changes what we think (e.g. we may think we like someone because we feel 'butterflies' in our stomach when we see them)
- Sensations and behaviours
  - Body sensations tell us about the environment, and can affect how we react to it (e.g. if my body is ready to fight or flight, I may react more aggressively to situations than if I am calm)
  - We can act in ways that influence our body (e.g. exercise may give us energy, deep breathing can help us relax...)

Facilitators may find it useful to focus the group on one connection at a time.

Activity 2 – A Recipe for Success

Once the young people have become confident in understanding and using the model, they may then fill in their own hot cross bun. Facilitators should encourage young people to consider a key difficulty or troubling situation which they encounter often (facilitators may refer to the child's goals or any difficulties which they have expressed in previous sessions). Young people may then break down their 'cycle' into the hot cross bun format. Young people may do this individually for 10-15 minutes, with facilitators providing additional support if needed.

Once the young people have completed their own forms, they can share them with the group. This may allow young people to support each other, particularly if they experience similar difficulties. Young people may then discuss possible strategies to break their cycle (think back to 'hot' and 'cold' strategies). This may include some of the strategies introduced in previous sessions (e.g. challenging thought biases, relaxation exercises...) or even new strategies that the young people come up with. Attendees may formulate these strategies into specific plans to try out in their own time.

Facilitators should tactfully question or redirect any unhelpful strategies suggested during this session. Facilitators should also take note of relevant difficulties, goals and plans, as these will be relevant in future sessions, where young people will be asked to reflect on their progress and make plans for how to maintain it after the group ends (e.g. sessions 7–8).

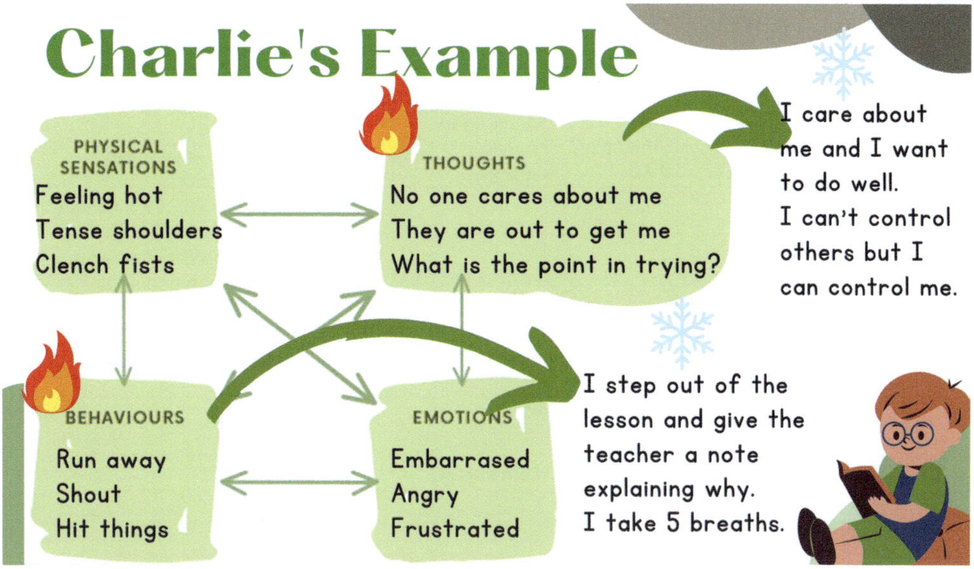

Figure 14.4

Task 3: Thought Diary Homework

Duration: *10 Minutes*
Objectives: *Promote revision and reflection*
Support attendees to challenge unhelpful thoughts and behaviours and recognise what maintains their 'cycle'
Resources: *Thought diary worksheets*

Following the explanation of the CBT cycle, facilitators should hand out the 'Thought Diary Worksheet'. Facilitators should explain that thought diaries allow us to track how the elements of the 'hot cross bun' (CBT model) affect our everyday lives. This can help the young people identify unhelpful thoughts or actions which maintain their problems. Furthermore, the use of a thought diary prompts the young people to reflect on these thoughts, and provides an opportunity for them to consider alternative strategies that may be more useful (e.g. challenging unhelpful biases, giving priority to more helpful thoughts and actions...). Overall, thought diaries promote the generalisation of skills learnt within the SHERBET sessions to the everyday lives of young people.

Research into CBT homework, such as Thought Diaries, has suggested that both the quantity and quality of the homework have an impact in the overall effectiveness of interventions (Rees et al., 2003[4]; Rees et al., 2005[5]). Those who complete the homework consistently and to a good standard tend to have a greater reduction in mental health symptoms (e.g. depression, anxiety).

Instructions on how to complete the diary are included in the worksheet. Young people may benefit from reading these alongside facilitators and completing an example entry as a group.

What happened? - Describe the situation - Where were you? - Who were you with?	Thoughts - Unhelpful thoughts - Helpful thoughts	Emotions - What were they? - Intensity? 0-10	Physical feelings - (e.g. stomach ache/heart beating quickly)	Behaviour - What did you do?	Could i have thought or done something differently? - Any thinking errors? - What will i change for next time? - What helped that i can use again?

Figure 14.5

Task 4: Object-Based Mindfulness and Relaxation

Duration: *5 Minutes*
Objectives: *Explore mindfulness*
Resources: *Speakers and recording OR prepared script*
Object (one for each attendee)

For this exercise, facilitators should provide a neutral object (i.e., not emotionally significant) for young people to focus on during the exercise. Some possible objects may include fidget toys, pencils, pens, cups... Alternatively, facilitators may ask young people to bring in an object for the purposes of this exercise.

Facilitators should explain (referring to the 'hot cross bun') that by engaging in this exercise (behaviour), we aim to relax our bodies (sensation) helping us feel more calm (emotion). In previous sessions we have used different kinds of mindfulness and relaxation exercises (e.g. breathing, music) to help us 'return to neutral'.

This particular mindfulness exercise involves an object. By focusing on the object through our senses (sight, smell, touch...) we can directly target the 'sensations' part of our hot cross bun. Some people prefer to use a smooth or fluffy object, as it is more pleasant to touch. However, the most important part of this exercise is practicing our attention, observation and relaxation skills, so any object will do!

It may be useful at this point to remind attendees of an appropriate non-verbal sign (e.g. putting their hand up) if they need a break from the exercise. This will allow participants to communicate any needs without disturbing others in the group.

Delivering Mindfulness Content

Facilitators should briefly cover what can be expected from the exercise:

- Attendees should be quiet and focused on their own objects. They may wish to sit further away from each other to make this easier.
- The mindfulness exercise will last approximately 5 minutes.
- Throughout the exercise, some questions will be asked about the objects in front of them. They should reply to these questions in their heads, not out loud.

- The aim of the exercise is to be relaxed but alert (not asleep!). Sitting comfortably may help with relaxation but young people should be encouraged to keep both feet on the ground.
- This exercise does not require attendees to close their eyes.

Facilitators may then deliver the mindfulness content. Facilitators should endeavour to maintain a relaxed tone, and allow for pauses in the delivery so young people may mentally engage with the content.

Alternatively, facilitators may select an appropriate recording of an object-based mindfulness or meditation exercise with an approximate duration of 5 minutes. It is essential for facilitators to listen to the selected recording in full, assessing its relevance and appropriateness, prior to sharing it with the young people.

Sample Script – Object Mindfulness

Find a comfortable position to sit in. We want to be relaxed but alert, we don't want to fall asleep. I find it helpful to keep both of my feet on the ground and my hands on my knees.

First start by relaxing your body and focusing on your breath.

Take a nice, full deep breath in...and breathe out.

Let your belly rise and fall with each breath, no need to do anything at all, just breathe.

Good.

During this exercise, you may notice your mind wandering. That is totally normal and completely okay. When you notice your mind becoming distracted, thinking of something other than what we are doing right now, just imagine yourself putting that thought on a little cloud, and watch it float away.

Now focus on the object in front of you. Look at it, but don't touch it yet.

We are going to really focus our attention on the object. Notice all its details without judgement. They are not good or bad, they just are.

Notice what you can see about the object. What colours does it have? What shapes does it have? What does the texture look like?

Change the object's angle slightly. Can you see anything new? Has the angle of the light changed on it?

Come back to your breath for a second, good job.

Now, you can touch the object. Touch the object and notice how it feels in your hands: are they soft, rough, cold, warm...?

Notice how different parts of the object have different textures and feels.

Good job.

Now let's take a couple more of deep breaths, in... and out...

As you breathe, keep looking around your object, focusing on every detail you can see, feel and touch.

With a final breath, open your eyes and come back to the room.

References

1 Beck, J. S., & Beck, A. T. (2011). *Cognitive behavior therapy: Basic and beyond.* Guilford.

2 Riise, E. N., Wergeland, G. J. H., Njardvik, U., & Öst, L. G. (2021). Cognitive behavior therapy for externalizing disorders in children and adolescents in routine clinical care: A systematic review and meta-analysis. *Clinical Psychology Review*, *83*, 101954.

3 Wergeland, G. J. H., Riise, E. N., & Öst, L. G. (2021). Cognitive behavior therapy for internalizing disorders in children and adolescents in routine clinical care: A systematic review and meta-analysis. *Clinical Psychology Review*, *83*, 101918.

4 Rees, C., McEvoy, P., Juniper, U., Nathan, P., & Smith, L. (2003). Mechanisms of change in CBT: Does homework matter?. In *Proceedings of the 38th APS Annual Conference* (pp. 179–183). The Australian Psychological Society Ltd.

5 Rees, C. S., McEvoy, P., & Nathan, P. R. (2005). Relationship between homework completion and outcome in cognitive behaviour therapy. *Cognitive Behaviour Therapy*, *34*(4), 242–247.

15 Session 7

Communicating with Others

Task 1: Check-In

Duration: 10 Minutes (+ Icebreaker duration)
Objectives: Promote peer support and reflection
Resources: None

Facilitators can prompt the attendees to reflect on the thought diary completed for homework. Some useful prompts may include:

- Describe a challenge which you wrote in your thought diary and how you used the diary to manage it.
- How did you find the thought diary? Was it helpful/unhelpful? Hard/easy?
- What were some challenges you faced when trying to complete the thought diary?
- What were some positives of using the thought diary?
- Do you think you would use the thought diary again in the future? Why/why not?

Facilitators should praise young people for their effort in using the diary, and highlight any positives which they observe in the attendees' feedback of the homework. Facilitators may find it useful to bring spare diaries for those young people who wish to continue practicing their use. It may also be useful to identify challenges which the young people encountered when using the diary, potentially creating adapted diaries for those attendees who need them.

This exercise also helps facilitators observe attendees' ability to remember and apply the information covered in sessions. Facilitators may support attendees to review any content which they are struggling with.

Task 2: The Ways We Communicate

Duration: 40 Minutes
Objectives: Learn about different communication styles
Reflect on non-verbal communication cues
Practice assertive communication
Resources: Character scripts OR relevant videos

Facilitators should explain that the focus of this session is going to be communication styles. They may assess the group's existing knowledge on the matter by asking them to shout out any communication styles they know.

DOI: 10.4324/9781003666738-15

Activity 1 – What Is Communication?

Some attendees may benefit from a review of the 'what is communication' activity in Session 3 of the SHERBET manual. This will test the knowledge of attendees and ensure that they are considering all the factors affecting the quality of communication, which they can apply to the communication styles.

Facilitators can encourage attendees to recall and name elements which affected communication. Facilitators may play a video or act out a conversation as an example for young people to unpick. As in Session 3, facilitators may remind attendees of any key elements which they may have missed.

Attendees may also share any experiences of communication or miscommunication which they have had since Session 3. This may produce useful examples and showcase attendees' skills in retaining and applying the content learned in sessions. Facilitators may wish to provide their own examples to role model session engagement as well as role model their skills in communication and reflection.

Information for Facilitators

Communication is essential for interacting with others, building relationships, resolving conflicts and achieving goals. However, as explored in Session 3, achieving good communication can be complicated. Session 3 explored some of the elements that may affect communication (e.g. mood, channel, other people...). This session aims to build on that understanding to help young people harness those elements into a style of communication that can help them achieve their goals whilst remaining respectful of others and their needs: Assertiveness.

However, before working on building assertiveness skills, it is important for young people to recognise the whole spectrum of communication styles. This will allow young people to reflect on how they currently communicate, identifying its impact and possible improvements. Additionally, a greater awareness of communication styles may allow attendees to recognise

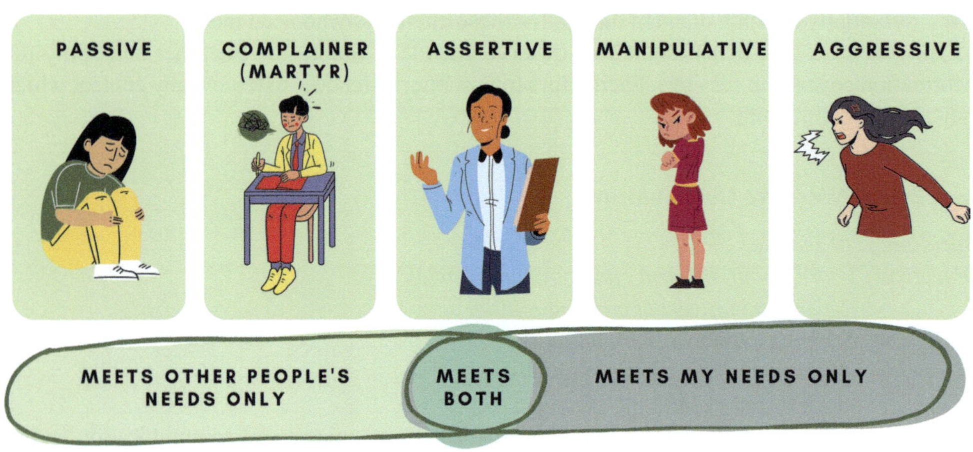

Figure 15.1

when they or someone else is adopting a particular style, therefore empowering them to change their approach to the conversation.

Awareness of communication styles, introspection into one's own communication style and assertiveness training have been linked to improved quality of communication[1, 2] and reduced difficulties with anger management.[3, 4] Additionally, assertiveness has been linked to emotion regulation skills[5], suggesting that targeting assertiveness may improve emotion regulation in young people.

Overall the main goals of improving assertive communication are:

- To improve the confidence and skill of young people when communicating their needs and goals, therefore increasing the likelihood of early and effective communication.
- To increase the likelihood that these needs and goals will be met, therefore reducing the number of stressful and straining situations for the child.
- To improve young people's skills when communicating after stress, strain or anger are already present.

Communication Styles Outlined

The present model outlines four main communication styles: Passive, aggressive, assertive and passive-aggressive (broken down into 'complainer' and 'manipulative' for ease of understanding).[6] This model may be simplified to 3 levels (Aggressive, Assertive and Passive)[7] to increase accessibility.

Passive

A passive individual will place the needs of others above their own. This is a dishonest communication style because the person does not share their thoughts, needs and emotions. If they do try to express disagreement this will be very soft-spoken and quiet and they will quickly take it back if not immediately supported.

Passive communicators are likely to speak quietly, have a 'small' posture (e.g. slouching) and make little eye contact*.

Passive communicators might therefore:

- Feel anxious, stressed or burned out because they have no control over their lives.
- Feel depressed or hopeless because they are 'stuck' in situations they don't want to be in.
- Feel confused and unsure of how to achieve the things they want or need.

Example

Brin has an English exam tomorrow and she wants to study for it. Brin's best friend, Dot, does not know about the exam. Dot asks Brin to help her with her homework. Brin says that she's not sure she can today. Dot says 'Please, you are so good at maths and I am so rubbish! Come on, best friend, you'd be doing me a huge favour'. Brin agrees and helps Dot with her homework. She is worrying about her exam the whole time they are working together but she doesn't say anything.

Passive-Aggressive

This term describes individuals who seem passive but are reacting in a subtle or indirect way. Multiple authors have broken passive-aggressiveness into a multitude of dimensions.[8] For the purposes of simplicity and promoting understanding the current model divides passive-aggressiveness into two main presentations: one which fulfills the needs of others (complainer) and one which fulfills the needs of the person (manipulative).

Complainer

Complainers may appear passive to others (e.g. quiet, agreeable, 'small' posture). Like passive communicators, they put others' needs above their own. However, complainers are more aware of the impact that being passive is having on them and feel more strongly about it, although they may struggle to accept this anger and frustration (e.g. 'I'm fine!'). This is a dishonest communication style because the person does not share their thoughts, needs and emotions with the right people (e.g. the source of the problem).

Complainers act passively in front of the person whose needs they are meeting (e.g. a teacher, a parent) and will complete the tasks. However, they might:

- Mutter to themselves instead of confronting the problem.
- Pretend like there is not a problem.
- Complain about the problem to others (e.g. friends) but do nothing about it.
- Hide how they feel by using facial expressions and posture, for example, smile when they are angry.

As a result of this behaviour, complainers might:

- Feel stuck and powerless.
- Become disconnected from those around them, for example, lose friends who are tired of the negative comments.
- Sometimes 'explode' with anger or frustration at the problem, often creating a different problem as a result.
- Sometimes 'explode' with anger or frustration at things that are not the problem, simply because they've kept in the feelings too long.

Example
Azan's classmate pronounces his name wrong. Azan finds this very annoying, and always complains to his friends about this classmate. When the classmate calls his name Azan will mutter under his breath 'For God's sake... every time...' but when the classmate asks 'What did you say? Sorry I didn't hear you'. Azan just smiles and says 'Nothing'. Azan's friends tell him to talk to his classmate and explain the situation but Azan keeps avoiding it and pretending everything is fine.

Manipulative

Manipulative communicators may appear passive to others (e.g. quiet, agreeable, 'small' posture). However, they are 'secretly' putting their own needs above those of others. This is a dishonest approach because they are not sharing their thoughts, needs and emotions. Instead, manipulative communicators will try to find 'roundabout' ways to achieve their goals, without caring if they are negatively impacting other people's needs, rights or wellbeing.

Manipulative communicators will superficially agree with others. They may appear co-operatively but secretly they are doing things that will achieve their own goals. This may include annoying, disrupting or hurting others. Manipulative communicators may hold onto grudges, pretending they have got over them, and will engage in sabotage and revenge.

As a result of these behaviours, manipulative communicators might...

- Become disconnected from those around them, for example, losing friends who realise the manipulation.
- Feel very alone and misunderstood.
- Feel weak and resentful because they are not actually fixing their problems.
- Not realise the impact of their actions on others, because they mainly think about their own goals and feelings.
- Sometimes 'explode' with anger and frustration at the problem, often creating a different problem as a result.

Example

Sofia is not doing well in science. She blames her science teacher and thinks that he must hate her. She has been spreading rumours in school about this science teacher, hoping they might get him in trouble. When the teacher asks her to do something in class she messes it up on purpose but pretends it's an accident (e.g. takes extra long to give the books out so class starts late).

Aggressive

Aggressive communicators put their own needs first, disregarding the needs, rights and well-being of others. This may result in the verbal or physical abuse of others. This is an inappropriately honest approach, because aggressive communicators do express their thoughts and needs but do so in a way that is hurtful to others.

Aggressive communicators will try to use a 'big' and intimidating posture (e.g. stand tall, stand too close, puff chest out). They will speak in a loud voice and might shout. They may use threats and humiliation to control others. They are likely to criticise, blame or attack others whilst taking little responsibility themselves. They tend to not listen well and will therefore interrupt and act impulsively.

As a result of these behaviours aggressive communicators might...

- Become disconnected from those around them, for example, people, even friends, may choose to avoid them.
- Feel very alone and misunderstood.
- Not realise the impact of their actions on others, because they mainly think about their own goals and feelings.
- React with anger and frustration at the problem, leading to more problems.
- Feel frustrated and unsure of how to achieve their goals because they struggle to accept responsibility.
- End up in dangerous or life-threatening situations, for example, if others also respond aggressively.

Example

McKenzie's friend (Theo) is on his phone and not listening. McKenzie is annoyed at Theo because he cancelled plans with other friends so they could hang out and now he feels bored and ignored. McKenzie shouts at Theo calling him a bad friend and he threatens to smash Theo's phone if he doesn't put it away right now.

Assertive

Assertiveness describes a style of communication which allows the person to achieve their goal or resolve a conflict whilst being perceived as appropriate and polite by the listener.[9]

Assertive people will be open and honest about their thoughts and needs whilst remaining respectful of others and their feelings. They will advocate for their rights and needs without imposing on the rights and needs of others.

Assertiveness looks like:

- Posture – stand/sit straight without attempting to make themselves big or intimidating.
- Tone of voice – talk in a confident tone of voice, for example, not shouting (aggressive) or whispering (passive).
- Eye contact – good, regular eye contact*.
- Facial expressions match the internal feelings.
- Timing the message – assertive communication is achieved best when a good time for the conversation is chosen. For example, both parties are calm, there is privacy and plenty of time to discuss the problem without other distractions/responsibilities.
- Content of the message – this is the most important element of assertive communication.[7] Nothing else matters if the final message delivered is too aggressive or passive. Assertive messages are clear and respectful. Communicators may start messages by expressing their feelings with 'I...' statements (e.g. I feel upset and embarrassed when you tell me off in front of the class). Any requests made will be specific and direct. Assertive communicators will also have thought about their requests before discussing them, making sure they are realistic and they respect others' needs.
- Listening – it is important to also listen to what others have to say. This helps communicators understand better the situation and the needs of others. This way assertive communicators can negotiate an outcome that meets everyone's needs.

As a result of assertive communication, these people might...

- Feel connected to others – they will understand how others feel and others will understand how they feel.
- Feel in control of their lives.
- Resolve their problems as they come up.
- Prevent problems from happening by communicating needs respectfully before they become a problem.
- Create a respectful environment where others also feel safe and can communicate well.

Example

Lucas has a diagnosis of ADHD. He is allowed to carry fidget toys in school and has a note for this. Lucas was told off in front of his whole class by Mr Porter for looking distracted with his fidget toy. Lucas felt very embarrassed and angry that this new teacher had told him off when he was allowed these toys. Lucas waited until break time, when he was a bit more calm and he had time to talk to Mr Porter 1:1. Lucas showed Mr Porter the note and explained that the toy helped and he was listening in the lesson, so he would want to keep using his fidget toys. Lucas also told Mr Porter that he felt very upset when Mr Porter told him off in front of everyone and asked Mr Porter to please talk to him at his desk instead of shouting from the front of the class. Mr Porter agreed to this. However, Mr Porter asked that, if Lucas wanted to use a fidget toy

during lessons he would have to use quiet ones (e.g. stress balls instead of poppers) because the sound could be distracting for Mr Porter and other students. They both agreed to this plan.
*Please note that some young people (e.g. Autism Spectrum Disorder,[10] Social Anxiety Disorder[11]) may struggle to establish and maintain what many consider appropriate eye contact. Facilitators should reassure students that eye contact is only one of the many features of communication and many people may struggle with it. These students may be encouraged to focus their skill-building on other elements of communication, for example, verbal communication.

Activity 2 – Communication Styles

After reviewing attendees' understanding of the elements affecting the quality and effectiveness of communication, facilitators may proceed to explaining some of the standard known communication styles.

Facilitators may first inquire if the attendees know any communication styles, which they can shout out. Facilitators should then present the above-described model. Given how well known the 'passive-aggressive' communication style can be, facilitators may find it useful to acknowledge its existence and clarify that it has been broken down into two sub-styles: 'complainer' and 'manipulative'.

To gain an initial understanding of the communication styles, facilitators should introduce these one at a time. It may be beneficial to encourage young people to suggest descriptions (e.g. posture, gestures, tone, message content) for each communication style before these are explained. This allows facilitators to observe pre-existing knowledge and attitudes of attendees. Facilitators may then add any necessary detail to the information provided by attendees.

Use of Videos: Facilitators may supplement the explanations of communications styles with video clips which demonstrate them. Alternatively, they may test young people's knowledge by playing different videos and asking young people to identify the communication style, as well as explain what 'clues' pointed them to the answer (e.g. posture, volume...). Some good examples of different styles of communication may be sourced from YouTube and television shows such as *Friends* or *The Office*.

Task 3: Emotion Charades and Roleplay

Duration: *20–25 Minutes*
Objectives: *Promote engagement*
Exploring accuracy when identifying others' emotions
Explore how accuracy may change depending on our emotions and experiences
Promote empathy and perspective taking
Resources: *Character scripts OR relevant videos*

Activity 1

Facilitators will provide scripts for the young people which give them emotions and a context for their characters. Sample scripts are provided in the manual. Facilitators may also request 'conflict' examples from relevant professionals working with the attendees (e.g. school staff) so the situations will be relevant to them. Facilitators should assign characters an 'unhelpful' communication style (not assertive).

The young people may then interact as their characters for a limited time period. The rest of the young people can observe the interaction (alternatively facilitators may break down the group into pairs who can run roleplays simultaneously).

**Note: Facilitators may use appropriate videos instead of roleplay. This may be beneficial for groups who are reluctant to roleplay or for 1:1 delivery.*

At the end of each roleplay exercise, facilitators should promote discussion amongst the young people. Some prompts may include:

- What communication style was each character using? How could you tell?
- Did the characters achieve their goals?
- How did character X feel? Why?
- How did the communication style affect the conversation? For example, was communication easier/harder and why?
- What would have been a better way for character X to approach the situation?

This exercise aims to make young people reflect on how their communication style may impact other people as well as their own goals[12,13]. For example, being on the receiving end of aggressive communication may help realise how their behaviour and communication style is perceived by others.

This exercise also aims to improve empathy and perspective taking by encouraging young people to view the situation through another person's eyes[14]. As noted in Session 3, role play has been widely and successfully used as a method of promoting empathy in a variety of samples, ranging from schoolchildren[15] to offenders.[16, 17] Increased empathy, in turn, results in a reduction of aggressive behaviour and improvements in compassion and conflict resolution.[18]

Activity 2

Attendees should then repeat the roleplays done in Activity 1 but, this time, all characters should aim to communicate assertively to resolve the conflict. Facilitators may pause roleplays at this stage to give feedback to attendees and redirect behaviours if these steer away from assertive communication.

Prior to carrying out the roleplays facilitators should explore with young people ways in which they can communicate assertively. One example includes the following sentence formula:

1. Name the feeling: This should be an I statement (as opposed to 'you made me feel' which is more accusatory): *'I felt upset and frustrated when'.*
2. Name the situation: *'When you complained to my sister that I had upset you, without telling me that I had upset you.'.*
3. Name the desired outcome: *'I would prefer if you approached me directly if I upset you, so it gives me a chance to learn and do better'.*
4. Let go out the outcome: Remember your circles of control, influence and concern. You can't control other people or situations, but you can control your own behaviour. If you become angry or controlling when people don't do as you'd like, you stop behaving in an assertive way.

Facilitators may also encourage young people to identify their own assertive sentence starters or sentence formulas.

At the end of each roleplay exercise, facilitators should again promote discussion amongst the young people. Some prompts may include:

- What did your character do to be assertive?
- What was character X thinking? Were these helpful thoughts (to maintain assertivity)?
- Did the characters achieve their goals?
- How did character X feel? Why?
- How did the communication style affect the conversation? For example, was communication easier/harder and why?
- Are there any improvements which character X could try next time there is a conflict?

Extension Activity: To further practice assertive communication, facilitators may prompt attendees to repeat the roleplay exercise but, this time, only one character is trying to be assertive. This aims to challenge attendees to remain assertive even when facing an 'unhelpful' communication style. It is important for attendees to be aware that, even if they communicate assertively, there may be situations where the other person is unreasonable. In these cases, they should endeavour to maintain an assertive and respectful approach, exiting the situation and finding alternative solutions if necessary.

Example
Lucas has a diagnosis of ADHD. He is allowed to carry fidget toys in school and has a note for this. Lucas was told off in front of his whole class by Mr Porter for looking distracted with his fidget toy. Lucas felt very embarrassed and angry that this new teacher had told him off when he was allowed these toys. Lucas waited until break time, when he was a bit more calm, and he had time to talk to Mr Porter 1:1. Lucas showed Mr Porter the note and explained that the toy helped and he was listening in the lesson, so he would want to keep using his fidget toys. Lucas also told Mr Porter that he felt very upset when Mr Porter told him off in front of everyone and asked Mr Porter to please talk to him at his desk instead of shouting from the front of the class. Mr Porter told Lucas that he didn't care about his little paper and he was not allowed fidget toys. When Lucas tried to assertively explain that this was agreed with the school, Mr Porter shouted at Lucas and said, 'Do not talk back to me!'. Lucas decided that Mr Porter was not going to listen so he said okay and left the room calmly. Lucas then spoke to other teachers he trusted about the situation. These teachers helped Lucas talk to the head-teacher who told off Mr Porter for not letting Lucas access his reasonable adaptations.

Maintaining Safety: The character scripts aim to showcase conflict between the characters, as well as possible poor communication. It is important throughout the exercise to maintain awareness of the following:

- Some people may have a history of traumatic experiences, and may be affected by the content in these scenarios. It is important during this exercise to monitor the young people and check-in if they seem uncomfortable or upset. Please refer to 'Dealing with difficult issues' for further guidance.
- It may be relevant to give a trigger warning prior to the exercise and encourage young people to speak up if they need a break or become upset (or remind them of the group agreements, if these cover the need for breaks and time-outs).
- It is important to prevent inappropriate use of the roleplay exercise. Create clear boundaries prior to the exercise and remind young people of the group agreements (e.g. respect). For

example, it may be useful to remind young people that, even though their character/emotion is angry, they cannot insult, hit or threaten their peers. Facilitators should be acutely aware of peer dynamics when selecting 'actors' for a scenario, and should intervene as soon as possible if they observe an 'actor' becoming overly intense in their behaviour (e.g. shouting, believable threats, invading personal space).

- 'Actors' may be encouraged to sit in a specific chair for their character. This can help facilitators maintain physical distance between actors to prevent invasions of personal space.
- It may also be appropriate to introduce a word or sign which actors can use to stop the roleplay if they become upset.

Task 4: Imagery-Based Mindfulness and Relaxation

Duration: *5 Minutes*
Objectives: *Explore mindfulness*
Resources: *Speakers and recording OR prepared script*

Facilitators should remind attendees (referring to the 'hot cross bun') that by engaging in this exercise (behaviour), we aim to relax out bodies (sensation) helping us feel more calm (emotion). In previous sessions we have used different kinds of mindfulness and relaxation exercises (e.g. breathing, music) to help us 'return to neutral'.

It may be useful at this point to remind attendees of an appropriate non-verbal sign (e.g. putting their hand up) if they need a break from the exercise. This will allow participants to communicate any needs without disturbing others in the group.

Delivering Mindfulness Content

Facilitators should briefly cover what can be expected from the exercise:

- Attendees should be quiet and focused on themselves. They may wish to sit further away from each other to make this easier.
- The mindfulness exercise will last approximately 5 minutes.
- Throughout the exercise, some questions will be asked about the images in their heads. They should reply to these questions in their heads, not out loud.
- The aim of the exercise is to be relaxed but alert (not asleep!). Sitting comfortably may help with relaxation but young people should be encouraged to keep both feet on the ground.
- This exercise does not require attendees to close their eyes.

Facilitators may then deliver the mindfulness content. Facilitators should endeavour to maintain a relaxed tone and allow for pauses in the delivery so young people may mentally engage with the content.

Alternatively, facilitators may select an appropriate recording of an object-based mindfulness or meditation exercise with an approximate duration of 5 minutes. It is essential for facilitators to listen to the selected recording in full, assessing its relevance and appropriateness, prior to sharing it with the young people.

Sample Script – Safe Place

Find a comfortable position to sit in. We want to be relaxed but alert, we don't want to fall asleep. I find it helpful to keep both of my feet on the ground and my hands on my knees.

First start by relaxing your body and focusing on your breath.
Take a nice, full deep breath in...and breathe out.
Let your belly rise and fall with each breath, no need to do anything at all, just breathe.
Good.
Think now of a place where you feel safe.
It could be anywhere you like such as the beach, or in your own room.
It could be an imaginary place, somewhere you have read about, somewhere that you have built in your mind.
I like to imagine myself in a small beach, quiet except for the sounds of the waves. I have made this place up in my mind so only I know where it is and what it looks like.
Picture all the details of your safe place: what you can see, smell, touch...
Look at all the colours around you. The shapes. The objects.
Good.
Take another deep breath in and imagine the smells around you in this safe and wonderful place.
Good job.
Now focus on the sensations – what can you feel in this place? For me, it is the sand beneath my feet and the sun on my face.
Now lets take a couple more of deep breaths, in... and out...
As you breathe, keep looking around your safe place, focusing on every detail you can see, smell, feel and touch.
Notice your body, relaxing. It is safe.
With a final breath, open your eyes and come back to the room.

References

1 Omura, M., Maguire, J., Levett-Jones, T., & Stone, T. E. (2017). The effectiveness of assertiveness communication training programs for healthcare professionals and students: A systematic review. *International Journal of Nursing Studies, 76*, 120–128.

2 Avşar, F., & Alkaya, S. A. (2017). The effectiveness of assertiveness training for school-aged children on bullying and assertiveness level. *Journal of Pediatric Nursing, 36*, 186–190.

3 Wilcox, D., & Dowrick, P. W. (1992). Anger management with adolescents. *Residential Treatment for Children & Youth, 9*(3), 29–39.

4 Dunbar, B. (2004). Anger management: A holistic approach. *Journal of the American Psychiatric Nurses Association, 10*(1), 16–23.

5 Allahyari, B., & Jenaabadi, H. (2015). The role of assertiveness and self-assertion in female high school students' emotional self-regulation. *Creative Education, 6*(14), 1616.

6 *The Four Basic Styles of Communication.* (2014). University of Kentuky Violence Intervention and Prevention Center. Retrieved 21 March 2022, from www.uky.edu/hr/sites/www.uky.edu.hr/files/wellness/images/Conf14_FourCommStyles.pdf.

7 Pipas, M. D., & Jaradat, M. (2010). Assertive communication skills. *Annales Universitatis Apulensis: Series Oeconomica, 12*(2), 649.

8 Johnson, N. J., & Klee, T. (2007). Passive-aggressive behavior and leadership styles in organizations. *Journal of Leadership & Organizational Studies, 14*(2), 130–142.

9 Mitamura, T. (2018). Developing the functional assertiveness scale: Measuring dimensions of objective effectiveness and pragmatic politeness. *Japanese Psychological Research, 60*(2), 99–110.

10 Senju, A., & Johnson, M. H. (2009). Atypical eye contact in autism: models, mechanisms and development. *Neuroscience & Biobehavioral Reviews, 33*(8), 1204–1214.

11 Schneier, F. R., Rodebaugh, T. L., Blanco, C., Lewin, H., & Liebowitz, M. R. (2011). Fear and avoidance of eye contact in social anxiety disorder. *Comprehensive Psychiatry, 52*(1), 81–87.

12 Tan, K., Wegmann, K., Patino, R., Hand, B., Mitchell, J., & Moser, K. (2021). Social and emotional learning group work during the COVID-19 Pandemic, the reopening, and the mobilization for racial justice. *Children & Schools*, *43*(2), 118–122.
13 Southam-Gerow, M. A. (2013). *Emotion regulation in children and adolescents: A practitioner's guide*. Guilford Press.
14 Weisz, E., & Zaki, J. (2017). Empathy building interventions: A review of existing work and suggestions for future directions. In *The Oxford Handbook of Compassion Science* (pp. 205–217).
15 Castillo, R., Salguero, J. M., Fernández-Berrocal, P., & Balluerka, N. (2013). Effects of an emotional intelligence intervention on aggression and empathy among adolescents. *Journal of Adolescence*, *36*(5), 883–892.
16 Pithers, W. D. (1999). Empathy: Definition, enhancement, and relevance to the treatment of sexual abusers. *Journal of Interpersonal Violence*, *14*(3), 257–284.
17 Webster, S. D., Bowers, L. E., Mann, R. E., & Marshall, W. L. (2005). Developing empathy in sexual offenders: The value of offence re-enactments. *Sexual Abuse: A Journal of Research and Treatment*, *17*(1), 63–77.
18 Klimecki, O. M. (2019). The role of empathy and compassion in conflict resolution. *Emotion Review*, *11*(4), 310–325.

16 Session 8

Moving Forward

Task 1: Check-In

Duration: *10 Minutes (+ Icebreaker duration)*
Objectives: *Promote peer support and reflection*
Resources: *None*

This final session aims to support attendees' reflections of the skills achieved so far. It also aims to build upon these skills, planning for future goals and challenges so that young people will not relapse into unhelpful strategies.

Facilitators may want to prompt the attendees to reflect on the content of the previous session:

- Last session we covered different styles of communication, can you say the name OR act out any of the styles?
- Have you noticed anyone in your life being one of the styles (passive, complainer, assertive, manipulative, aggressive...)? Can you describe what happened (how did you recognise the style, how it made you feel, how you responded)?
- Tell me about a time that you were assertive this past week.

Or prompt them to reflect that this is the last session in the program:

- What is one helpful thing that you have learned in these sessions? Why is it helpful?
- What is something that you thought we would cover but we haven't yet?
- What is something that is still unclear or you want to learn more about?
- Tell me one good change that you have made since we started sessions.

These questions may allow facilitators to identify knowledge and skills which the young people need to cover or review prior to the end of the group. They also prompt young people to reflect on the positive changes they have achieved. By focusing on the changes achieved and the changes they wish to achieve, young people are likely to show improved motivation, self-efficacy[1] and overall outcomes.[2]

DOI: 10.4324/9781003666738-16

Task 2: Revising the Emotion Thermometer

Duration: *35 Minutes*
Objectives: *Promote peer support and reflection*
Create comprehensive and relevant emotion thermometers
Promote a collaborative approach to emotion regulation and behaviour management
Resources: *Previously completed emotion thermometers (+Blank copies)*

Information for Facilitators

This exercise aims to update the existing Emotion Thermometers, reviewing accuracy and adding details to ensure they are comprehensive and relevant to the needs of young people. This worksheet, once completed, aims to fulfil the role of a Positive Behaviour Support (PBS) plan[3], as described in Session 3.

The completed emotion thermometers should be shared (with the consent of attendees) with key stakeholders in the young person's environment (e.g. school staff, parents) to promote a wide and consistent use of the plan.

Activity Information

Facilitators should provide printed copies of the already-completed emotion thermometers for the young people. Young people should then be prompted to reflect on the following:

- **Coping with the emotion** – The last time we reviewed the thermometers young people were prompted to rate at which level (out of 10) they felt:
  - I feel 'out of control'.
  - I feel uncomfortable and struggle to manage the emotion.
  - I can manage the emotion.

  Attendees should review this and explore if their tolerance of the emotion has changed (e.g. before I felt out of control at a 6/10 but now I can manage up to an 8/10, although I still struggle to control myself from a 5/10).
- **Reading the signs** – Young people should review the warning signs and behaviours which they described at each level of intensity, checking that they are still accurate. Young people may have increased their awareness for behaviours and warning signs since they last completed the worksheet, so this may be an appropriate time to add detail to the worksheet.
- **Adding strategies** – Young people should review the strategies which they included at each level of intensity. They may wish to reflect on which strategies have been helpful or unhelpful so far, removing unhelpful ones. They may also want to add any strategies they have gained since the last time they completed the worksheet.
- **Reviewing triggers** – Young people may also benefit from reviewing the potential triggers for a sudden escalation of emotion, adding newly identified triggers and eliminating irrelevant ones.
- **Consent for sharing** – Facilitators should promote the sharing of this tool with key stakeholders in the young person's like (e.g. school staff, family). They should explain the benefits of having others understand what triggers and what helps the behaviour, so they may better support the young people. Facilitators should also highlight the communication

function of thermometers, as young people could use them as a tool to explain how they are feeling and what they need. If consent is obtained, facilitators may then share the tool with relevant individuals. Facilitators may also encourage young people to explain the tool to these stakeholders, so they may solidify their understanding and ownership of the tool.

Task 3: Hope for the Best, Plan for the Worst

Duration: *25 Minutes*
Objectives: *Promote peer support and reflection*
Promote reflection and preparation for future challenges
Resources: *None*

This exercise prompts attendees to identify potentially challenging situations which they may face (e.g. being told off, a difficult conversation, an upcoming exam...). Facilitators should encourage young people to identify at least one situation each.

Once the potentially triggering situations are identified, these may be presented one by one to the group. The young person will then be encouraged to make a plan on how they want to handle the situation. The young person should consider:

1. **What** is the **situation**? Who, what, where…
2. Goal: **What** do I **want** to **achieve**? What do I want or need?
3. How do I want to achieve my goal?
   - **What** do I want to **say**?
   - **How** do I want to **say** it?
   - **When** do I want to **say** it?
4. What **challenges** might come up?
   - Getting angry or upset
   - Getting interrupted
   - The other person disagreeing…
5. **How** can I **overcome** them?
   - Strategies…
   - Help from others…

Young people may also be prompted to consider what the consequences might be for the behaviours and messages they plan on using.

The young person may then make a plan for how to tackle the situation so they can obtain a favourable outcome whilst avoiding the use of challenging behaviours. They can share this plan with the group.

Peers and facilitators may provide feedback and support for the young person's plan. If the young person is struggling with the plan, peers may provide helpful suggestions. It may be also useful to challenge unhelpful or unrealistic plans. Attendees should be reminded of the consequences of their actions (e.g. you may want to shout, but what do you think will happen after? Will you get told off or punished?).

These scenarios may be shared with the group via narrative presentation (i.e. talking about it). They may also be acted out in the form of a role-play, so attendees can rehearse their communication and emotion regulation skills within the session. Peers or facilitators can support with the role play (i.e. be the other character) or observe and provide feedback.

Task 4: Closure

Duration: *15 Minutes*
Objectives: *Promote peer support and reflection*
Support closure of the group setting
Resources: *Remember your strengths worksheet*

In this final group session it is essential for facilitators to support attendees in the group closure. Facilitators should help attendees to let go of the group whilst still maintaining the skills and experiences they have gained from it.

The end of a group, like many other changes, can elicit feelings of anxiety and uncertainty. This may contribute to unhelpful reactions from group members, such as denial (e.g. 'forgetting' repeatedly the end date), regression (e.g. sliding back into the behaviours that led them to the group) or reactivity (e.g. fight or flight, becoming aggressive or dropping out early).[4] A more appropriate response may be 'reviewing' where participants reminisce of group experiences, which can help them prepare to let go.

As noted by Robb (2022), 'Learning how to say goodbye is a skill in itself' (p.135), and group members have not always had previous experiences of ending relationships in a positive and healthy manner.[5]

Closure Strategies

One way in which facilitators can support attendees with the emotional separation of the group is to allow them to work though their separation anxieties. Facilitators may encourage attendees to reflect on what things they appreciated and resented within the group. This allows attendees to reflect a balanced account and work through unresolved emotions.

Although it is important to validate the feelings of attendees, facilitators should aim to not appear punitive or rejecting of any group members. Benson (2002) advises 'I find the simplest way of working with such behaviour is to describe what is happening and wonder aloud what is behind it. Members are usually able to verbalize and reflect on their motives quite quickly' (p.162).[4]

Facilitators can also support attendees with practical aspects of ending the group. For example, attendees may wish to consider and plan for a specific time every day/week where they can reflect on their emotions and progress with their goal. This way they can continue to hold space for themselves, their feelings and their progress, as opposed to completely losing this practice after the end of the group.

Attendees may also benefit from identifying people with whom they can discuss topics similar to those covered in the group (e.g. emotions, goals, worries). This way they can have access to a reliable support network which they can reach out to when the group is no longer available.

Another way in which facilitators can support the closure of the group is by prompting discussion of the progress and changes that have been achieved in the group. Attendees may wish to reflect on where they were at the start, where they are now and where they wish to be in the future. This places the group within the context of their lives as something that has contributed to their development but is only a small part of their experience. It reframes the group closure, turning it from an ending to the beginning of something else.

Most notably, the end of the group should be accompanied by a celebration of achievement and a show of gratitude. Facilitators may wish to bring in treats or games for this.

Overall, the closure of each group may vary depending on the needs or expressed wishes of attendees (e.g. some attendees may want to 'celebrate' by bringing cake or playing a ball game). Facilitators are encouraged to review the strategies and select which are most appropriate for their group's needs. Nonetheless, some sample questions and a sample activity have been provided for reference.

Sample Discussion Prompts

- Share with the group something you enjoyed and something you didn't like in the group.
- Are there any people you can talk to about the things we have covered in this group (e.g. emotions, anger, strategies...)?
- Do you feel closer to your goal than when we started? Why/why not?
- What is something that you can do after the group ends so you can keep getting closer to your goal?
- What is something impressive that you did/achieved in the group?
- What is something you are looking forward to once the group ends?

Facilitators should encourage young people to provide written responses for the following (see 'Reviewing Achievements' worksheet):

- The most important things that I have learned in SHERBET:
- Something I have learned or realised in SHERBET that I do not want to forget (e.g. coping skills, something helpful/unhelpful I do...):
- Something I did well/achieved in SHERBET:

Sample Activity

Each attendee should be given a sheet of paper upon which they write their name. This paper sheet is then passed around to the person on their left, who has to write a kind comment or a compliment about the person whose sheet it is. This is repeated until every attendee's sheet has been written in by all their peers. Attendees then can read these comments either in private or out loud for the group to hear.

This exercise aims to promote positive feedback between peers as well as positive reflections of the group. Additionally, the written format allows attendees to keep these positive comments as a memento of the group.

Please note that facilitators must review all the pages before they are handed back to their owners, to prevent negative or unhelpful comments from being written. If facilitators suspect that this is likely to happen within their group, due to existing group dynamics, they should avoid this exercise.

References

1 Copeland, L., McNamara, R., Kelson, M., & Simpson, S. (2015). Mechanisms of change within motivational interviewing in relation to health behaviors outcomes: A systematic review. *Patient Education and Counseling*, *98*(4), 401–411.
2 Apodaca, T. R., & Longabaugh, R. (2009). Mechanisms of change in motivational interviewing: A review and preliminary evaluation of the evidence. *Addiction*, *104*(5), 705–715.
3 Allen, D. (2009). Positive behavioural support as a service system for people with challenging behaviour. *Psychiatry*, *8*(10), 408–412.
4 Benson, J. (2002). Work at the ending stage of the group: Separation issues. In *Working more creatively with groups* (pp. 155–164). Routledge.
5 Robb, M. A. (2022). Ending stage. In *Group art therapy*, edited by M. A. Robb (pp. 135–140). Routledge.

17 Maintaining Skills

This program endeavours to promote the generalisation and maintenance of the skills obtained throughout its duration. Throughout this program, attendees will have obtained knowledge and skills in emotion recognition, emotion regulation, empathy, communication and more.

The program structure promotes the initial application of these skills beyond the session through homework that prompts attendees to review and apply the knowledge between sessions. The structure also promotes maintenance of skills and knowledge by incorporating 'revision' tasks at the start of each session, whereby attendees can be tested on the content covered so they can practice recalling the content they remember and can be supported to review the content they forgot.

Facilitators can also promote the long-term impact of the program by encouraging young people to practice their skills between sessions. They may encourage young people to share positive uses of the knowledge, or even highlight positive uses that they may have observed in attendees. By highlighting and praising progress, facilitators may improve attendees' motivation and self-efficacy to continue applying the skills and creating positive change.

Collaborating agencies may also support the generalisation and maintenance of skills throughout the program delivery. Key stakeholders may be informed of attendees' progress and skills, so they may encourage their use outside of sessions. For example, 'Emotion Thermometers' may be shared with school staff or family members, so they may recognise the child's emotion intensity and provide more effective support by promoting the use of the helpful strategies described.

Completer's Workbook

In order to promote maintenance of skills in the long term, this program includes a completer's workbook, which synthesises the content of the program. The workbook contains sections on content covered (e.g. thought biases, communication), as well as activities completed (e.g. 'coat of arms').

In order to be most effective, workbooks should be personalised to each child's responses throughout the program (e.g. 'goals' and 'emotion thermometer' worksheets). As attendees complete and hand in worksheets, facilitators should transpose them to the final workbook. This way, attendees may review and apply the work they have completed. For example, by having access to the completed 'emotion thermometer' participants can revisit helpful strategies. Attendees may use the workbooks as a reminder of the knowledge and skills gained, as well as a visual guide for their continued application.

DOI: 10.4324/9781003666738-17

Workbooks may also be shared with key stakeholders in the young person's environment (e.g. school staff, parents). Promoting their awareness and involvement in the maintenance of skills can be highly effective:

- They may be aware of the existence of the workbook and related skills, therefore being able to promote its use amongst attendees.
- They may be aware of triggers and unhelpful strategies, therefore being less likely to contribute to an escalation of emotion and behaviour.
- They may be aware of helpful strategies, therefore being more effective in supporting the young person's emotions regulation and behaviour management.
- Awareness of tools included in the workbook (e.g. emotion thermometer) may also ease communication with the young people, as these tools can act as a visual communication platform (e.g. young people can point to how they feel and what they need).

These workbooks may also be updated as needed. Young people may wish to adapt the content of their worksheets to better reflect the triggers and skills as these evolve. In this way, the workbooks may maintain their relevance and usefulness for the young person's emotion regulation in a long-term capacity.

18 Worksheets and Resources

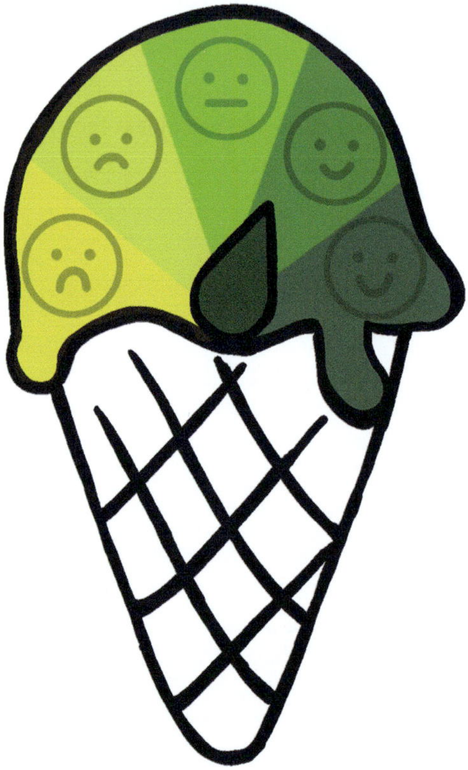

Figure 18.1

DOI: 10.4324/9781003666738-18

Service-Level Information and Agreement

> All of us experience emotions – negative, positive and everything in between. They are a part of our everyday lives. However, for some people, feeling these emotions can seem overwhelming, like an out-of-control roller coaster. Adolescents are particularly vulnerable to experiencing emotions in this way. This feeling of being overwhelmed emotionally can lead to a deep need to do something that will stop the intensity. This can lead to unhealthy coping strategies and risky or challenging behaviours.
>
> SHERBET Manual

The purpose of this intervention is to support young people with managing or regulating strong emotions when they feel overwhelming. The intervention is aimed at young people who may be presenting with poor emotional regulation. This may be seen through aggressive or impulsive behaviours.

What SHERBET Will Provide

The intervention consists of 12 sessions. This includes the following:

- Two group testing sessions (30 min each) – By having an assessment session at the beginning and end of the program we will be able to measure any changes in the young people and thus the effectiveness of the program.
  - The first group testing session will either be accompanied or preceded by a group information session where the young people will be informed of the purpose and structure of the group. This information session will also give young people a space to ask questions
  - The collection of this data allows facilitators to evaluate the effectiveness of the program. Additionally, an overall comparison of initial group scores and final group scores may be facilitated for the host organisation to observe the overall change achieved by the intervention.
- Two individual interviews (30 min each) with each young person participating in the group, one at the beginning and one at the end.
  - It may be possible to adapt these to a group format. However, the feasibility of each format will be decided by facilitators.
  - The final individual session will explore any remaining needs which the young people may have, and facilitate information for additional support if needed.
- Eight group sessions (90 min each including a small break)

We aim to deliver the sessions twice a week (week 1: assessment and interviews, weeks 2–5: group sessions, week 6: assessment and interviews), as this allows most groups to be delivered within one school term. This aims to promote long-term learning by having multiple, regular contacts with students and preventing long pauses in the program. However, it is possible to review the format to support a once-weekly session if this is required. It is expected that groups may have small breaks (e.g. half-term). During this time group sessions would also pause.

SHERBET facilitators aim to promote a collaborative and communicative approach. As a result:

- **Regular communications**: This will be encouraged to inform the host organisation of overall group progress – the designated 'link' member of staff may attend a short debrief contact after sessions to be aware of any key developments. There may be times where in-person contact may not be possible, in which case an email update may be sent.
- **Support with risk-related needs**: Facilitators will also communicate with host organisations if any significant risk issues arise, and collaborate with the management of these.
  For example, if a young person discloses self-harm, weekly check-ins need to take place to monitor the risk. This task may be taken on by facilitators or by an adequate member of staff (e.g. if the young person receives regular 1:1 support). If a member of staff agrees to do the weekly check-in (question content can be facilitated), facilitators will provide support and guidance with how to carry out the check-ins and can be contacted to provide support if any increases in risk are observed.
- **Appropriate notice:** If any significant changes need to occur to the group (e.g. re-scheduling a session, terminating a young person's participation…) facilitators will aim to openly communicate, involve relevant host-organisation staff in these choices and provide adequate notice and support for any changes.
- **Summary of outcomes**: At the end of the intervention, facilitators will meet with the host organisation to provide an overall summary of the group and its outcomes.

What the 'Host Organisation' Will Provide

- **Referrals for group participants**: The host organisation is expected to complete and send referrals for the SHERBET group via the usual referrals channel. Host organisations may consider the following:
  Service Factors
  - Number of participants: Host organisations may aim for around 6-8 participants in a group. However, this may be discussed with facilitators.
  - Referral detail: Even if we are expecting a referral and we have informally agreed to their participation on the group, it is expected that the referral form will outline the needs and difficulties of the young person. This allows our referrals team to approve and allocate the referral.
  - No double contacts: Young people will not be eligible for participation in SHERBET if they are already open to support from the delivery provider. If there is still a need for support after the completion of the current intervention, they may be referred for future groups.

  Participant Factors
  - Needs of participants: The needs of participants should be relevant to the purpose of the group. Further detail on the aims of the group is provided in the information sheet but we cover difficulties with: anger, impulsivity, difficulty managing emotions and other relevant difficulties.
  - Age of participants: Although mixed-age groups can be facilitated, we would recommend avoiding large age gaps, as the communication needs of participants may be too different to accommodate within the same group.
  - Group dynamics: The group setting requires participants to feel safe and be able to collaborate. Although we do tackle interpersonal conflict as part of our sessions, pre-existing conflicts may prevent attendees to engage with the content, and create an uncomfortable environment. This may result in a less effective intervention. We encourage host organisations to consider group dynamics when choosing group participants. If severely unhelpful dynamics are observed in the group (e.g. causing concern for the physical or psychological safety of any participants) we may have to discuss with the host organisation the need to take key participants out of the group (alternative support may be discussed).
- An appropriately sized **room for the sessions** to take place:
  - Depending on the expected needs of the group, it may be useful to consider a good 'time out' space for young people to take a break from the group session when needed.
- An **allocated member of staff** for SHERBET-related communications: This staff member will be the 'link' to the SHERBET group – they will be the main point of contact for any SHERBET communications (e.g. session debriefs, changes…).
  - Depending on the needs of the group, it may be appropriate for a member of staff to sit in the group sessions to support behaviour management. They may be, at times, asked to engage in exercises to promote attendee engagement.

- **Protected time for sessions**: An appropriate time for sessions to take place will be agreed with the host organisation. The host organisation should provide a full commitment to maintaining this protected time, and any changes (e.g. session cancellation, child taken out of session for an appropriate reason) should be communicated to facilitators with adequate notice.
    - Involving facilitators in these conversations will allow them to provide support and flexibility, when this is possible (e.g. if a child needs to be taken out of the session, facilitators may end the session 10 minutes early, as opposed to having the child leave mid-session to attend their other appointment).
- **Clear communication**: As mentioned throughout, clear communication with SHERBET facilitators will allow us to provide better support to the needs of the attendees.
- **Overview over the group progress**: A senior member of staff is encouraged to attend the start and end of intervention meetings. This will allow the host organisation to be appropriately informed of overall progress and will facilitate collaboration if any changes are needed.

This document aims to provide an in-depth explanation of what may be expected by facilitators and host organisations when delivering SHERBET. These aim to improve the quality of the intervention, collaboration between services and overall experience and effectiveness of SHERBET.

In signing this document both facilitators and host organisation staff agree:

- That facilitators and host organisation staff both understand the content of this document.
- That host organisation staff have had the chance to ask questions about the document.
- That host organisation staff have had the chance to discuss any difficulties that they may have adhering to this agreement, and reasonable adaptations have been discussed, and the document has been adapted accordingly.
- That both facilitators and staff agree with the contents of the document and will adhere to the roles and responsibilities which it outlines.

______________________	______________________
Sherbet Facilitator(s)	Host Organisation Staff

SHERBET Group Report

Participants and Attendance

Areas to cover:

- Number of students in the group
- Age and gender of cohort
- Attendance of participants.

Example:
This group is comprised of 5 participants (4 male, 1 female) ages 12-13. For the initial assessment and goal setting workshops, 2 participants attended both sessions and 3 attended only one of the workshops. Out of the 8 content-focused sessions 3 participants attended all sessions, 1 participant attended 7/8 and 1 participant attended 6/8.

Overall Engagement

Areas to cover:

- Quality of attendee engagement.
- Key observations regarding overall group functioning. For example, therapeutic bond, group dynamics, development of skills and insight…
- Key elements which affected engagement. Include beneficial strategies and why they were beneficial. For example, traffic light system for communicating the need for a 'time out'.

Example:
On the whole, participants have shown positive engagement in sessions, which has developed as sessions progressed. Some key observations throughout the group include:

Different needs: *Some participants engage better in spoken activities, whereas others engage better in written format or non-verbal engagement (e.g. standing in different areas of the room to show responses). A mix of delivery-styles for activities has been beneficial to promote engagement in all.*

Use of rewards: *Participants suggested having an outdoors break so they could play football. This has been a useful motivator to engage and has provided a brilliant space for participants to interact and co-operate.*

Group dynamics: *Overall participants have been respectful of one another. When individuals have shared difficult experiences, others have reacted appropriately and respectfully. There have been some tensions due to a member of the group taking over the conversation at times, distracting from the topic at hand; when deciding the group rules all attendees noted that staying on task and allowing everyone to have a turn to speak were shows of respect that they wanted in the group rules. These tensions have at times led to other members of the group making indirect comments. However, attendees responded to feedback – about both the comments and taking over conversations, which restored a good group climate. Most importantly, attendees have been able to remain respectful towards each other. They have shown an ability to regulate their* *comments and respond kindly to others, as opposed to impulsively reacting as they might have done in the past (e.g. saying something offensive).*

Self-reflection: *Attendees have shown good improvements in their ability to reflect on their behaviours and how they affect others and themselves. They have applied this in sessions, for example, communicating respectfully, using traffic light cards appropriately, recognising their triggers and difficulties. However, attendees often have more harsh and negative perspectives of their behaviour than facilitators, meaning that they may not always see their own improvements if these are not highlighted.*

Traffic light system: *Attendees were offered a traffic light system to communicate their inner feelings. This allowed facilitators to adapt and support as needed. Participants used this effectively, at times taking a break from the session to calm down before returning. We believe this was useful for preventing escalation within sessions which may have led to conflict. Feedback from school staff supporting the young people, as well as the young people themselves, showcase this as a useful tool, and young people were always happy to return to the session after using their 'red' light.*

Points for Development and Adaptations

Areas to cover:

- Discuss challenges faced, their impact and how they were handled

Example:
Boundary pushing*: There have been multiple occasions where attendees have had limited engagement and have continued pushing boundaries (e.g. putting heads on the table, using phones, not contributing, not paying attention) despite facilitator prompts. To some degree this is expected amongst the target population. However, the level of disruption it caused in two of the sessions meant it required direct addressing with the young people, as well as some session adaptations.*

- *Attendees' behaviour was addressed with them the following session. Emotion regulation and communication skills were role-modelled by highlighting that it wasn't best to have this discussion when attendees were still disruptive and upset, instead raising it at a time where they were calmer so they could actually listen and make a plan for it not to happen again. Both times students have been receptive to this and have shown insight into the way their behaviour impacts the session, facilitators and their peers.*
- *Group agreements were reviewed regularly and a copy was kept available to serve as a visual reminder for attendees of what was expected of them.*
- *To promote positive change and prevent defensive responses (e.g. closing off) facilitators accompanied the negative feedback with some positive feedback. This aimed to highlight attendees' strengths and improve their attitudes and beliefs about change (i.e. they often felt change was unachievable or out of their control).*
- *The traffic light system was amended to limit the spaces that young people could go to when using their red card (i.e. so they cannot wander around). 1:1 check-ins were also incorporated to address the problems and needs before they escalated (e.g. if an attendee*

looked disengaged or upset). This was highly effective and greatly improved quick recovery of mood and resulting engagement.

Organisation Support

Areas to cover:

- How the organisation has contributed and collaborated with SHERBET
- Positive areas and areas for development
- Highlight particular staff who have supported SHERBET, how they have done it and the impact this had

Example:
Initial Meeting: *From the initial meeting the school has shown a positive interest in the group. The school has shown great awareness of possible challenges which may be faced whilst running the group and have supported facilitators with them (e.g. choosing group members who will work well together).*
Ms X *has consistently provided invaluable contributions to the delivery of SHERBET.*

- *Supporting facilitators with introductions to the young people.*
- *Supporting facilitators with the use of rooms for assessments (simultaneous group and 1:1 sessions).*
- *Encouraging young people: Ms X has had a consistent and powerful impact on young people's attitudes towards SHERBET. She has promoted a view that SHERBET is a wonderful opportunity which the young people have been granted, out of everyone in the school. She instilled a sense of importance and pride about the group that certainly influenced attendees' attitudes and engagement.*

Overall having a designated member of staff to support with SHERBET has eased communication and organisation, resulting in much more effective delivery. Most importantly, Ms X's unique commitment and contributions to the group have significantly improved student engagement, facilitator satisfaction and overall quality of SHERBET.

Future Steps

Areas to cover:

- Any continuing support for students
- Useful resources which school may use to maintain group gains
- Key observations which may be of importance to the organisation

Example:
SHERBET aims to upskill young people to improve their emotion regulation and resulting behaviours. However, throughout the program we have also identified some information and resources which may be of use for the school.

- *Support beyond SHERBET: At the end of the group facilitators will assess the remaining needs of young people and, in collaboration with them, decide the best next steps. In this occasion, some attendees requested follow-up support (e.g. to complete content of sessions they had missed), which was arranged.*

- *Emotion thermometers: All attendees have completed an 'emotion thermometer' highlighting triggers, warning signs and helpful skills at different levels of their 'problem emotion' (e.g. anger). All attendees said they were happy to share these with staff. These may be useful to inform the school's approach to the behaviour management of these students. The forms may also be added to and edited as the needs and skills of young people change.*
- *Lunch time: Some students have routinely mentioned not having lunch/sufficient lunch (e.g. got distracted playing football). This impacted their mood and engagement in sessions. It may be useful for the school to consider this as a factor affecting the behaviour of students.*

Attendee Feedback

Areas to cover:

- Self-reported progress on their goals
- Favourite session/exercise
- Useful tools or skills gained in SHERBET
- Areas of improvement

Example:
Reflection on Goals – What goals did they wish to achieve through the group? How have they progressed towards them? This is what attendees responded:

- *I wanted to get in less trouble. It's going alright – I am getting less detentions, but I still have more warnings. This is for stupid things like talking, rocking on my chair… But my anger is better.*
- *I feel like my anger has got better. I would shout at teachers and get detentions. I think this is because of SHERBET. They have helped me to think about how I speak to people and what I want to achieve from conversations with them – shouting is not always the best, particularly with staff.*
- *I wanted to get less distracted, less zoning out, less restless. In SHERBET I have improved my concentration. I find this hard in other lessons.*
- *I wanted to control my anger so I can get a job in the future. I feel my anger has got a bit better. I have had no detentions. I have not got as angry.*

What was your favourite session?

- *The emotion thermometer – it helped me reflect on how I was feeling and how to make myself feel better.*
- *I liked the communication lessons with the videos.*
- *I liked that when we got a question right we got a gummy. I liked being competitive and thinking quickly.*
- *I liked the last session because we were all talking together – it was really nice.*
- *Acting out situations – this was funny and I liked joining in with everyone.*

What is something you found helpful?

- *The traffic lights helped me to easily communicate if I needed a break. It was a quick way to show what I needed.*
- *I liked having people to talk to about how I'm feeling.*
- *I liked the small group. It gave me a chance to get close to them.*
- *Everything was helpful, it was very good.*

What is something you didn't like?

- *I didn't like having to miss a lesson that is important to me. I would have liked to be in the group more but I did not want to miss this lesson.*
- *I wouldn't change any content.*
- *I didn't not like anything – it was all fine and I have enjoyed it a lot.*

Facilitators should thank the school at the end of the report (e.g. 'Thank you very much for your support so far. We hope that we can continue this collaboration') and provide their name and contact information.
Writing guidance:

- Please be aware of confidentiality throughout the report. Avoid naming attendees or revealing identifying information without their consent.
- Be aware that attendees may read this report. Ensure you are using respectful, considerate and trauma-informed language throughout.
- Be mindful of the language used when feeding back areas of development for the school and the students. Promote a compassionate and constructive approach.

Staff Debrief

This form should be completed by group facilitators immediately after the group session. This will allow you to identify significant topics for the session write-up and supervision meetings.

Session Number:
Session Title:
Number of Attendees:
Staff Present at Debrief:

Overall participant involvement and impressions – How did the session go?

Were there any significant comments or developments from participants?

Any group dynamics worth noting (i.e. how participants interacted with each other)?

Facilitator reflection – What went particularly well? What needs improvements?

What things will you repeat or change as a result?

Risk and safeguarding concerns (if any) and how they will be addressed:

Behavior and Feelings Survey – Youth Measure

How much have you had each of the following problems during the past week? Use a 0 to 4 scale. 0 = not a problem 4 = a very big problem	
My Thoughts and Feelings	Rating (0-4)
1. I feel sad	
2. I feel bad about myself, or don't like myself	
3. I feel down or depressed	
4. I feel nervous or afraid	
5. I worry about bad things happening	
6. I think sad or scary thoughts over and over again	
Internalising Problems Score:	
My Conduct and Behavior	Rating (0–4)
7. I talk back or argue with my parents or other adults	
8. I refuse to do what adults tell me to do	
9. I do things I am not supposed to do	
10. I am rude or disrespectful to people	
11. I argue with people	
12. I break rules at home or at school	
Externalising problems score:	
Total score	

Weisz, J. R., Vaughn-Coaxum, R. A., Evans, S. C., Thomassin, K., Hersh, J. Lee, E. H., Ng, M. Y., Lau, N., Raftery-Helmer, J. N., & Mair, P. (2019). Efficient monitoring of treatment response during youth psychotherapy: Development and psychometrics of the behavior and feelings survey. *Journal of Clinical Child and Adolescent Psychology*. Advance online publication.

Behavior and Feelings Survey – Caregiver Measure

How much has your child had each of the following problems during the past week? Use a 0 to 4 scale. 0 = not a problem 4 = a very big problem	
Thoughts and Feelings	Rating (0–4)
1. Feeling sad	
2. Feeling bad about himself/herself, or not liking himself/herself	
3. Feeling down or depressed	
4. Feeling nervous or afraid	
5. Worrying about bad things happening	
6. Thinking sad or scary thoughts over and over again	
Internalising problems score:	
Conduct and behaviour	Rating (0–4)
7. Talking back or arguing with parents or other adults	
8. Refusing to do what adults tell him/her to do	
9. Doing things he/she is not supposed to do	
10. Being rude or disrespectful to people	
11. Arguing with people	
12. Breaking rules at home or at school	
Externalising problems score:	
Total score	

Weisz, J. R., Vaughn-Coaxum, R. A., Evans, S. C., Thomassin, K., Hersh, J. Lee, E. H., Ng, M. Y., Lau, N., Raftery-Helmer, J. N., & Mair, P. (2019). Efficient monitoring of treatment response during youth psychotherapy: Development and psychometrics of the behavior and feelings survey. *Journal of Clinical Child and Adolescent Psychology*. Advance online publication.

Difficulties in Emotion Regulation Scale – 18 Item Version (DERS-18)

Instructions: Please indicate how often the following statements apply to you by selecting the appropriate option for each item.

1. I pay attention to how I feel.

1 Almost never (0–10%)	2 Sometimes (11–35%)	3 About half the time (36–65%)	4 Most of the time (66–90%)	5 Always (91–100%)

2. I have no idea how I am feeling.

1 Almost never (0–10%)	2 Sometimes (11–35%)	3 About half the time (36–65%)	4 Most of the time (66–90%)	5 Always (91–100%)

3. I have difficulty making sense out of my feelings.

1 Almost never (0–10%)	2 Sometimes (11–35%)	3 About half the time (36–65%)	4 Most of the time (66–90%)	5 Always (91–100%

4. I am attentive to my feelings.

1 Almost never (0–10%)	2 Sometimes (11–35%)	3 About half the time (36–65%)	4 Most of the time (66–90%)	5 Always (91–100%)

5. I am confused about how I feel.

1 Almost never (0–10%)	2 Sometimes (11–35%)	3 About half the time (36–65%)	4 Most of the time (66–90%)	5 Always (91–100%)

6. When I'm upset, I acknowledge my emotions.

1 Almost never (0–10%)	2 Sometimes (11–35%)	3 About half the time (36–65%)	4 Most of the time (66–90%)	5 Always (91–100%)

7. When I'm upset, I become embarrassed for feeling that way.

1 Almost never (0–10%)	2 Sometimes (11–35%)	3 About half the time (36–65%)	4 Most of the time (66–90%)	5 Always (91–100%)

8. When I'm upset, I have difficulty getting work done.

1 Almost never (0–10%)	2 Sometimes (11–35%)	3 About half the time (36–65%)	4 Most of the time (66–90%)	5 Always (91–100%)

9. When I'm upset, I become out of control.

1 Almost never (0–10%)	2 Sometimes (11–35%)	3 About half the time (36–65%)	4 Most of the time (66–90%)	5 Always (91–100%)

10. When I'm upset, I believe that I will remain that way for a long time.

1 Almost Never (0–10%)	2 Sometimes (11–35%)	3 About half the time (36–65%)	4 Most of the time (66–90%)	5 Always (91–100%)

11. When I'm upset, I believe that I'll end up feeling very depressed.

1 Almost never (0–10%)	2 Sometimes (11–35%)	3 About half the time (36–65%)	4 Most of the time (66–90%)	5 Always (91–100%)

12. When I'm upset, I have difficulty focusing on other things.

1 Almost never (0–10%)	2 Sometimes (11–35%)	3 About half the time (36–65%)	4 Most of the time (66–90%)	5 Always (91–100%)

13. When I'm upset, I feel ashamed with myself for feeling that way.

1 Almost never (0–10%)	2 Sometimes (11–35%)	3 About half the time (36–65%)	4 Most of the time (66–90%)	5 Always (91–100%)

14. When I'm upset, I feel guilty for feeling that way.

1 Almost never (0–10%)	2 Sometimes (11–35%)	3 About half the time (36–65%)	4 Most of the time (66–90%)	5 Always (91–100%)

15. When I'm upset, I have difficulty concentrating.

1 Almost never (0–10%)	2 Sometimes (11–35%)	3 About half the time (36–65%)	4 Most of the time (66–90%)	5 Always (91–100%)

16. When I'm upset, I have difficulty controlling my behaviors.

1 Almost never (0–10%)	2 Sometimes (11–35%)	3 About half the time (36–65%)	4 Most of the time (66–90%)	5 Always (91–100%)

17. When I'm upset, I believe that wallowing in it is all I can do.

1 Almost never (0–10%)	2 Sometimes (11–35%)	3 About half the time (36–65%)	4 Most of the time (66–90%)	5 Always (91–100%)

18. When I'm upset, I lose control over my behaviours.

1 Almost never (0–10%)	2 Sometimes (11–35%)	3 About half the time (36–65%)	4 Most of the time (66–90%)	5 Always (91–100%)

Original DERS (36 item) Citation: Gratz, K. L., & Roemer, L. (2004). Multidimensional assessment of emotion regulation and dysregulation: Development, factor structure, and initial validation of the difficulties in emotion regulation scale. Journal of Psychopathology and Behavioral Assessment, 26(1), 41-54.

DERS-18 (18 item) Holder: Springer Science+Business Media New York
Year: 2016

DERS-18 Hand Scoring

1. Reverse-code the following items using this scale:

1 = 5   2 = 4   3 = 3   4 = 2   5 = 1

Item	*Original Score*	*Reverse-Coded Score*
1. I pay attention to how I feel		
4. I am attentive to my feelings		
6. When I'm upset, I acknowledge my emotions		

2. Sum items for each subscale below. Note that for items with an asterisk (*), the reverse-coded score should be used (see right-hand column in the following table).

Awareness	*Clarity*	*Goals*
Item #1 * =	Item #2 =	Item #8 =
Item #4 * =	Item #3 =	Item #12 =
Item #6 * =	Item #5 =	Item #15 =
SUM =	SUM =	SUM =
Impulse	*Nonacceptance*	*Strategies*
Item #9 =	Item #7 =	Item #10 =
Item #16 =	Item #13 =	Item #11 =
Item #18 =	Item #14 =	Item #17 =
SUM =	SUM =	SUM =

3. To calculate the total score, sum the subscale scores in the following table.

Awareness	Clarity	Goals	Impulse	Nonacceptance	Strategies	Total score
+	+	+	+	+	=	

Original DERS (36 item) Citation: Gratz, K. L., & Roemer, L. (2004). Multidimensional assessment of emotion regulation and dysregulation: Development, factor structure, and initial validation of the difficulties in emotion regulation scale. Journal of Psychopathology and Behavioral Assessment, 26(1), 41-54.

Host Organisation Feedback Sheet

Thank you for your participation in the S.H.E.R.B.E.T programme. In order to continue assessing and improving our intervention, we would like to ask your school a few questions.

It is preferable if individual feedback is provided for each individual.

Feedback on Attendees

Attendee Initials	*Primary difficulties which the young person faced/ reason for referral to the SHERBET group*	*Intensity and severity of behaviours at time of referral (x/ 10)*	*Intensity and severity of behaviours after group completion (x/10)*	*Significant changes in the young person's emotional and behavioural difficulties since their involvement in SHERBET*

Feedback on SHERBET

Please provide feedback on the functioning of SHERBET and our facilitators:

1. It was reasonably easy for the organisation to host the SHERBET group (i.e. practical considerations: room, timings…).

Strongly disagree	Somewhat disagree	Neutral	Somewhat agree	Strongly agree

2. The amount of time and work required from the organisation and their staff was appropriate.

Strongly disagree	Somewhat disagree	Neutral	Somewhat agree	Strongly agree

3. The amount of time and work required from attendees was appropriate.

Strongly disagree	Somewhat disagree	Neutral	Somewhat agree	Strongly agree

4. Facilitators were collaborative and communicative with the organisation (e.g. designated SHERBET link staff).

Strongly disagree	Somewhat disagree	Neutral	Somewhat agree	Strongly agree

5. The description of SHERBET's purpose and objectives matched the observed outcomes.

Strongly disagree	Somewhat disagree	Neutral	Somewhat agree	Strongly agree

6. SHERBET provided sufficient support and resources for staff to assist participants beyond the duration of the group (e.g. maintenance of skills).

Strongly disagree	Somewhat disagree	Neutral	Somewhat agree	Strongly agree

7. SHERBET has areas that could be improved.

Strongly disagree	Somewhat disagree	Neutral	Somewhat agree	Strongly agree

What changes and improvements would you like to see in SHERBET in the future?

Any other feedback?

'Which… Are You?' Icebreaker

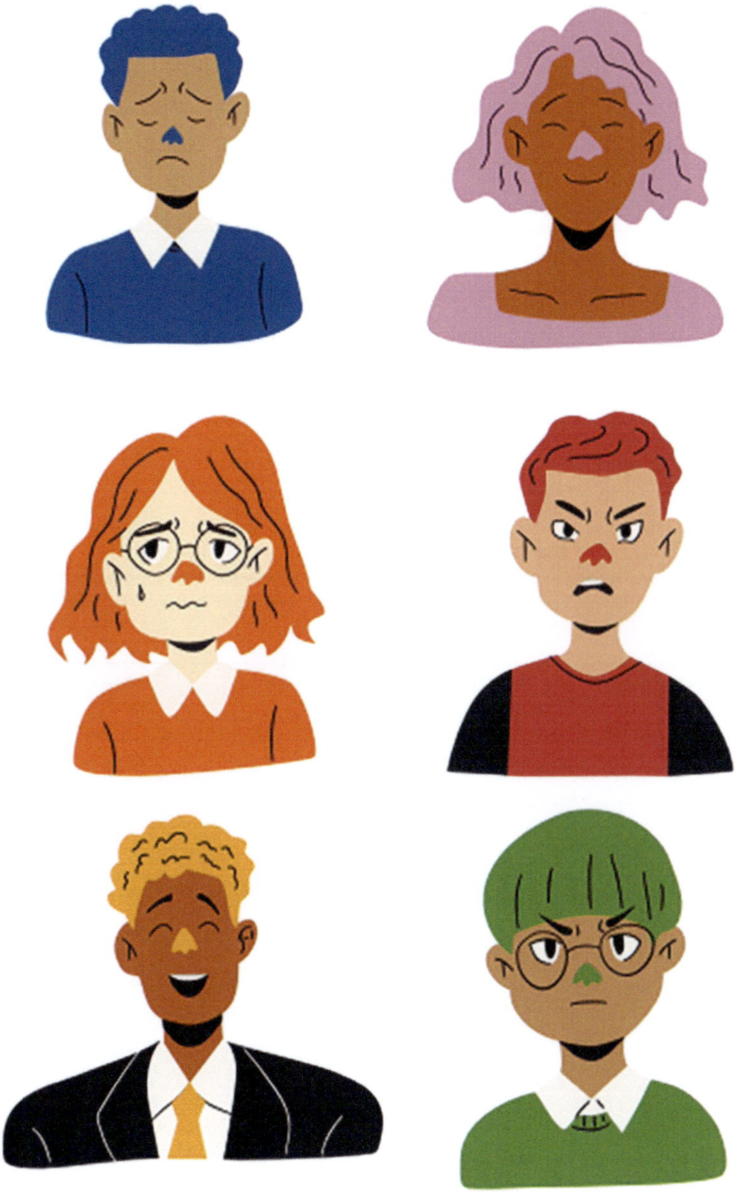

Figure 18.2

Human Bingo Icebreaker

Find someone who…

Has a pet	**Speaks another language**	**Has been to another country**
Plays football	**Has a sibling**	**Has a games console**
Helped someone out in the last week	**Has an allergy**	**Can whistle**

Traffic Light Communications

Some facilitators may benefit from introducing the 'traffic light' system for attendees to communicate when they are feeling distressed, overwhelmed or they need a break from the session. The specific meaning of each traffic light colour may vary depending on group agreements and the needs of young people. For example:

- Green: I am feeling okay to take part.
- Orange: I just need a minute (e.g. I can listen and be in the room but I'm not ready to take part in discussions).
- Red: I need a 5-minute break from the session.

Nonetheless, a blank template for the traffic lights is provided.

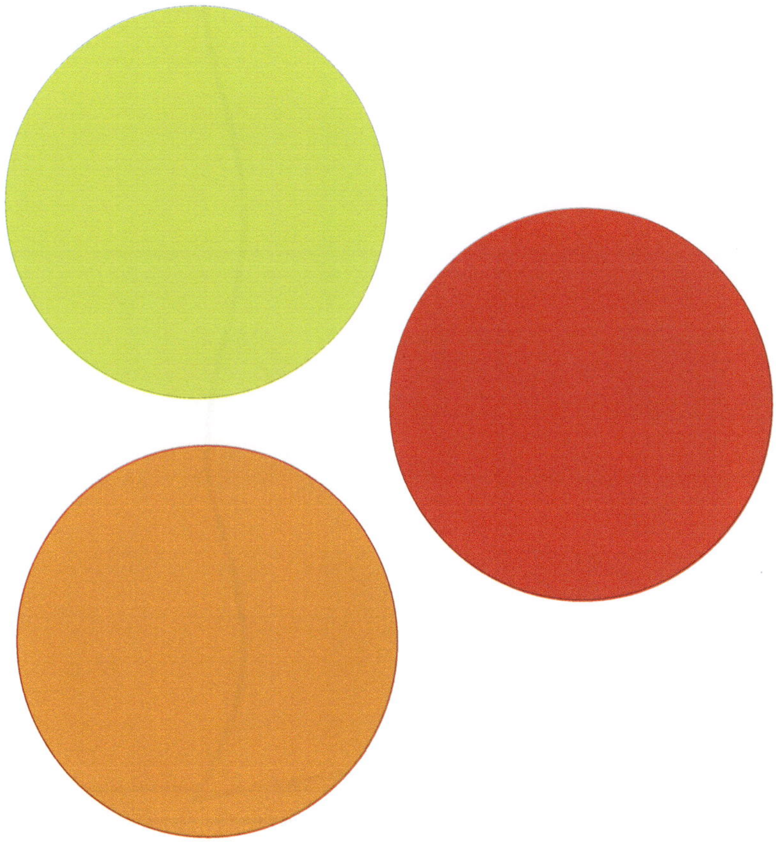

Figure 18.3

Flag of Me Icebreaker

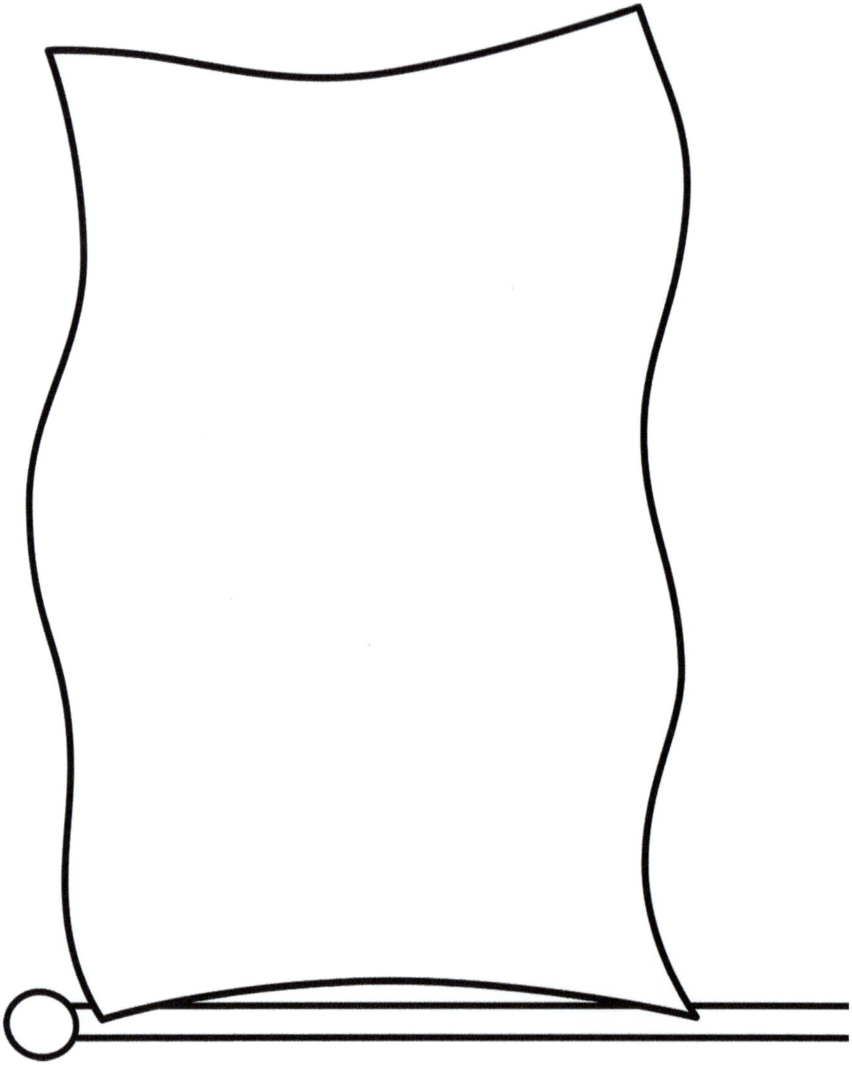

Figure 18.4

Information Leaflet

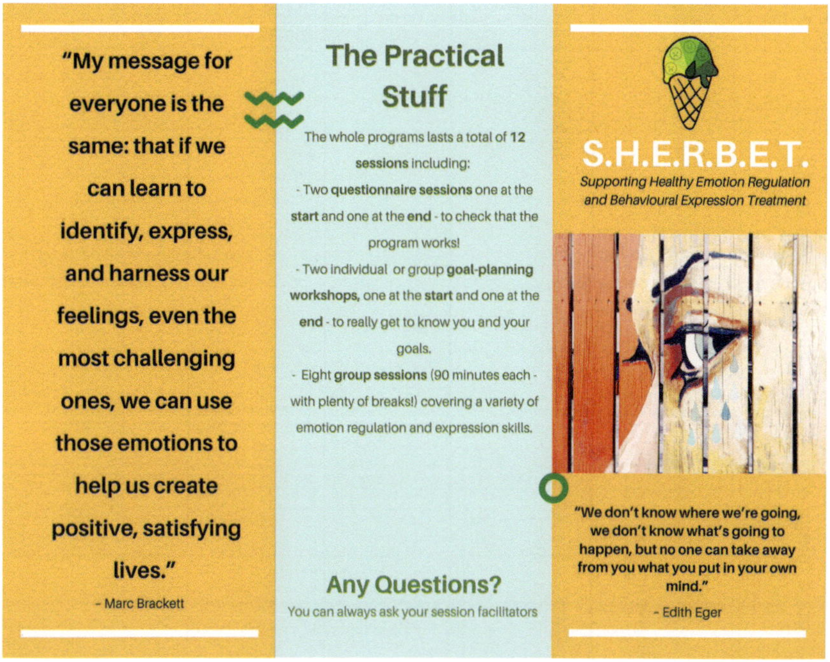

Figure 18.5

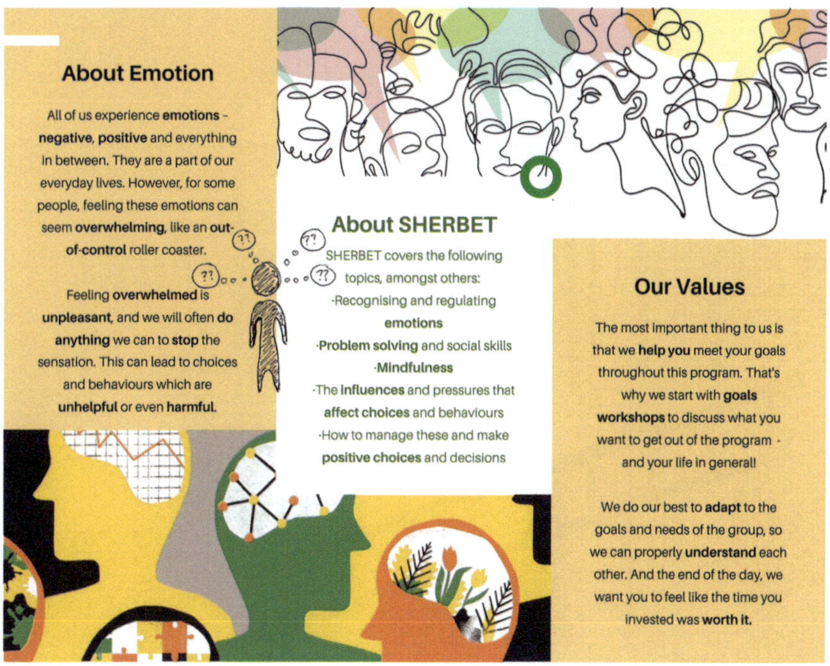
About Emotion
All of us experience emotions - negative, positive and everything in between. They are a part of our everyday lives. However, for some people, feeling these emotions can seem overwhelming, like an out-of-control roller coaster.
Feeling overwhelmed is unpleasant, and we will often do anything we can to stop the sensation. This can lead to choices and behaviours which are unhelpful or even harmful.
About SHERBET
SHERBET covers the following topics, amongst others:
·Recognising and regulating emotions
·Problem solving and social skills
·Mindfulness
·The influences and pressures that affect choices and behaviours
·How to manage these and make positive choices and decisions
Our Values
The most important thing to us is that we help you meet your goals throughout this program. That's why we start with goals workshops to discuss what you want to get out of the program - and your life in general!
We do our best to adapt to the goals and needs of the group, so we can properly understand each other. And the end of the day, we want you to feel like the time you invested was worth it.

Figure 18.6

Goal Setting Worksheet

NAME: Steps for Change

NAME:

Steps for Change

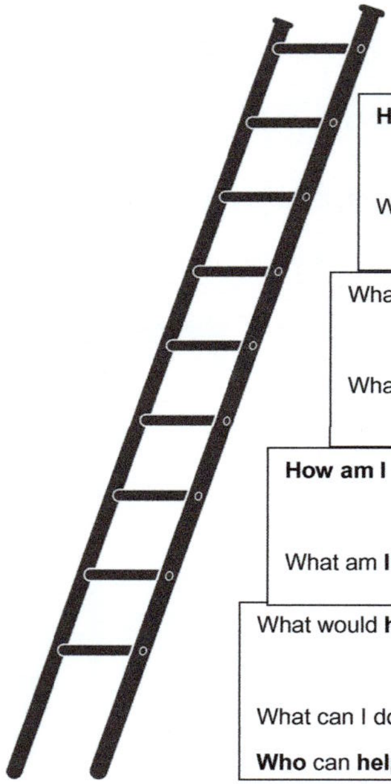

My Goal:

What **good things** will I get **from achieving my goal?**

How do I know I **achieved** my Goal?

What things may I **learn** in the program that can **help me achieve** my goal?

What do **I want** to **achieve** in this first step?

What things do **I need** to **do** to achieve it?

How am I now? Where am I in relation to my goal?

What am **I doing about it now**?

What would **happen** if I got **worse**?

What can I do if **I struggle** to achieve my goal?

Who can **help** me?

Figure 18.14.1

Ecological Model and Circles of Influence Worksheet

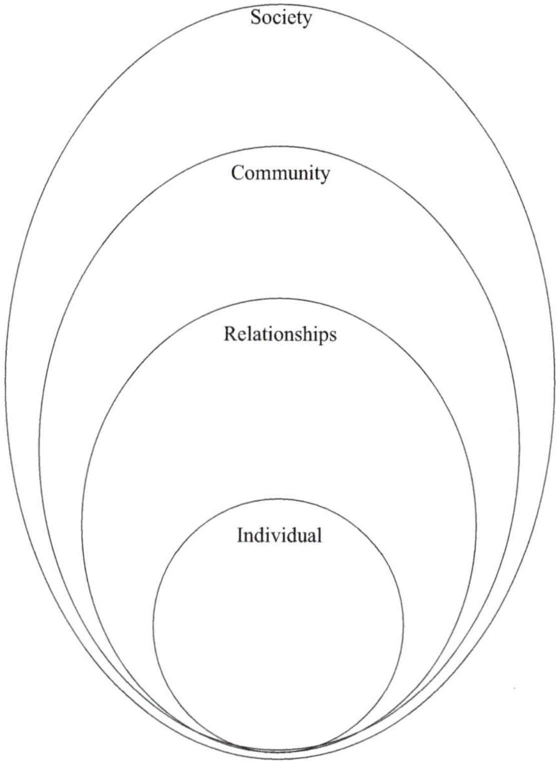

Activity 1

- **Look** at the **list of influences**. **Which** ones **influence your life**?
- **Write** them on the **diagram** above.
- Parents
- Extended Family
- Mental Health
- School
- History
- Friends
- Culture
- Knowledge
- Girlfriend/Boyfriend/Partner
- Laws
- Mass Media (TV, newspapers, news websites)
- Personality
- Social Media
- Siblings
- Neighbourhood

Are there any **other influences** in your life **not included** here?

Influencing Life

We need to **focus** our **energies** on what we **can control** and **influence!**

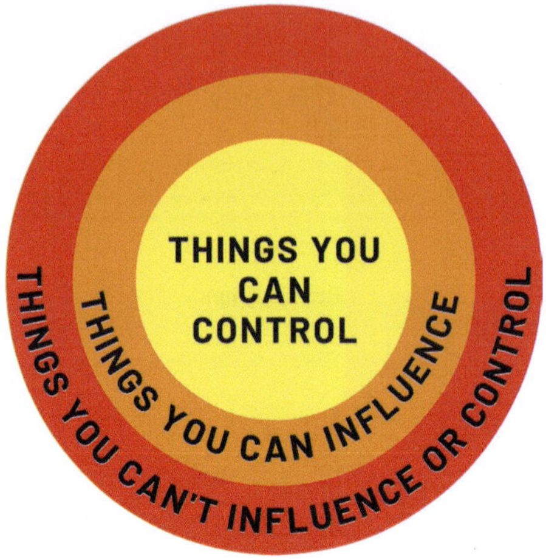

Figure 18.7

1. CIRCLE OF **CONTROL:** What we can **directly control**
2. CIRCLE OF **INFLUENCE:** The **worries** that we **can do something about**
3. CIRCLE OF **CONCERN:** Wide range of **worries** which **we cannot change** right now

Activity 2

- How do these **circles look** on **your 'Influences** in life'?
- **Draw them** on top
- What areas do you feel you **can control** or **influence**?

Reflection

- **What** do you **do** when **something happens** that **you can't control?**

Ecological Model and Circles of Influence Prompts

The World Around Us – *Resource Sheet*

SCHOOL 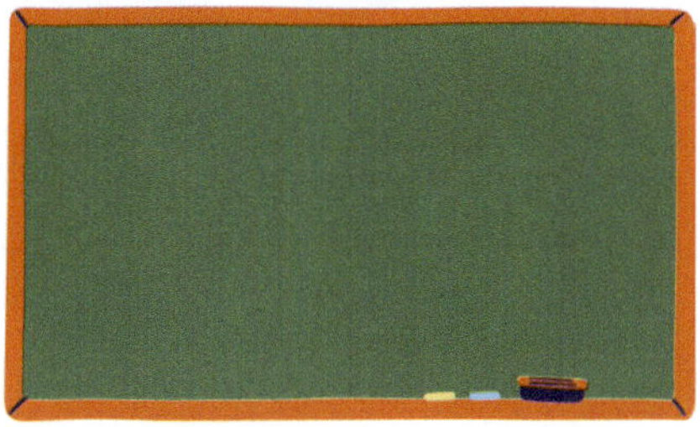 *Figure 18.16.1*	POLICE 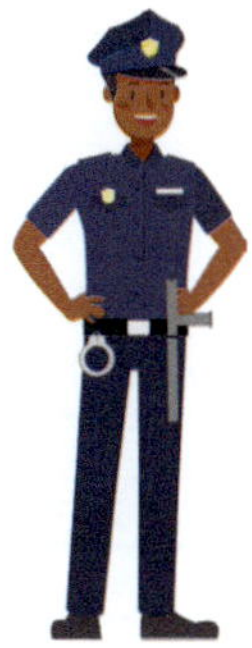 *Figure 18.16.2*
PARENTS/ CARERS 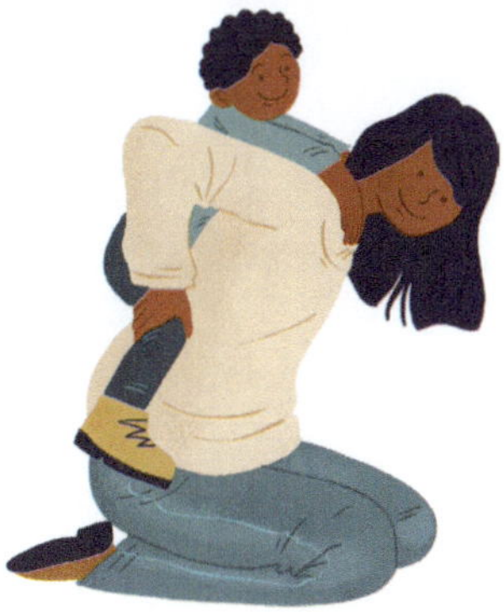 *Figure 18.16.3*	GOVERNMENT 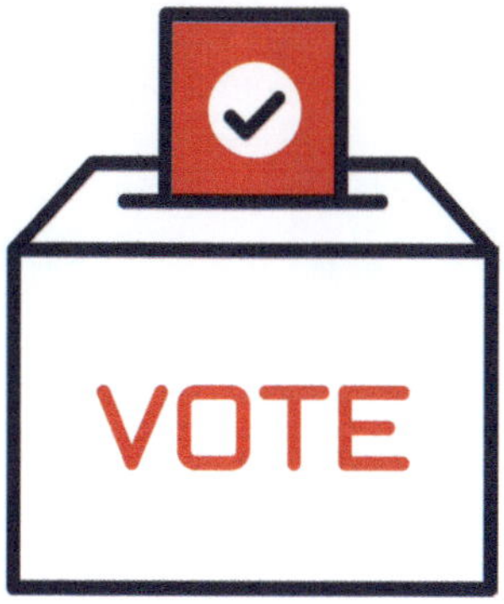 *Figure 18.16.4*

MEDIA

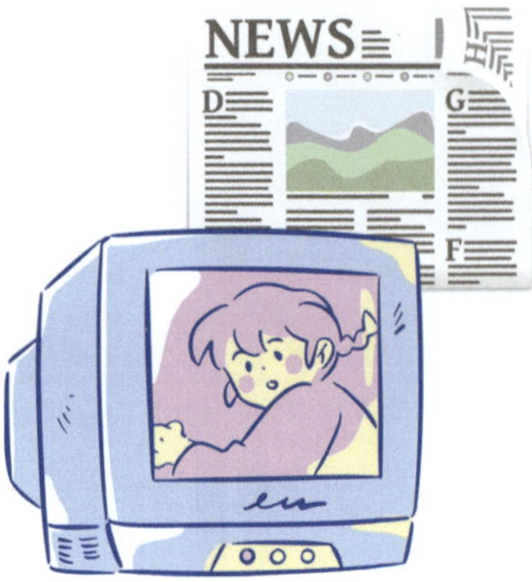

Figure 18.16.5

SOCIAL MEDIA

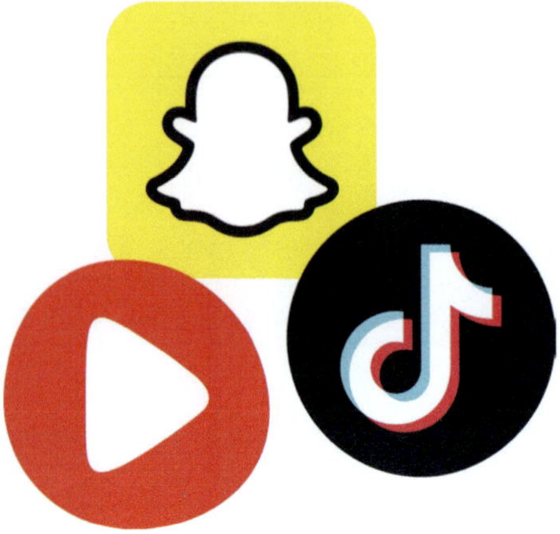

Figure 18.16.6

YOUNG PEOPLE

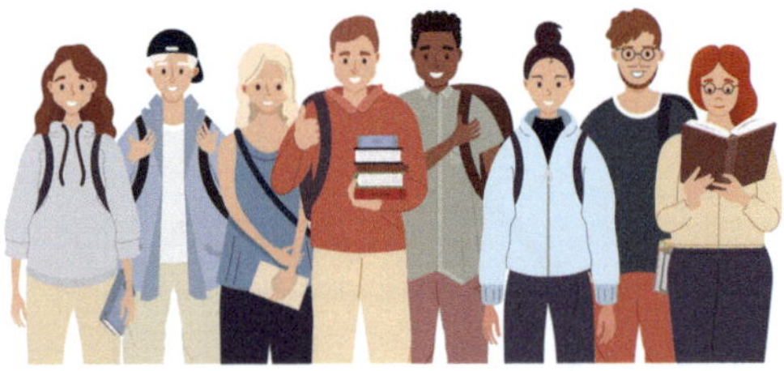

Figure 18.16.7

FRIENDS

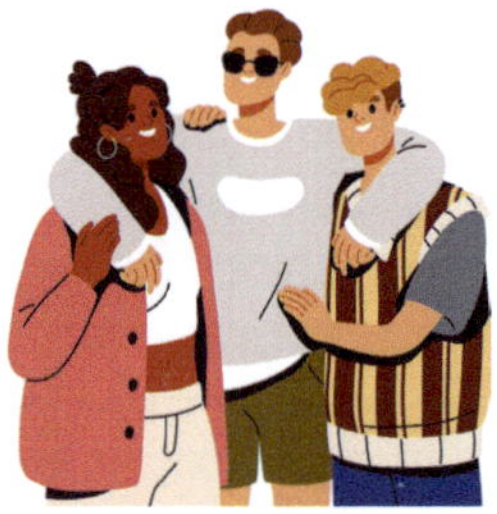

Figure 18.16.8

HISTORY

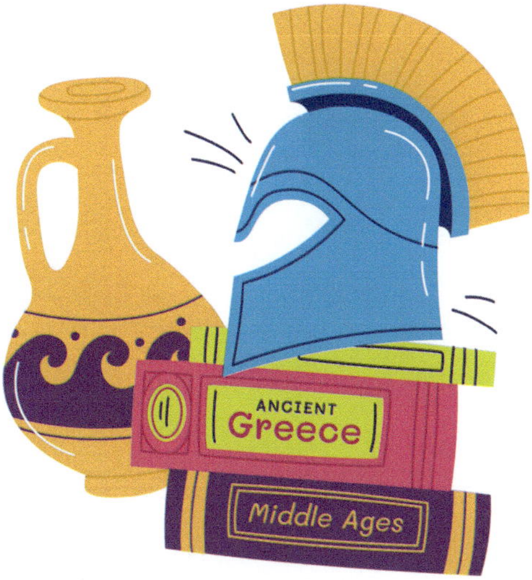

Figure 18.16.9

CULTURE

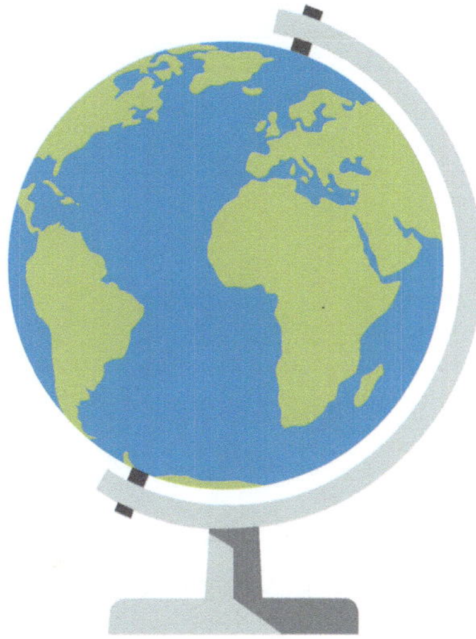

Figure 18.16.10

LAWS

Figure 18.16.11

NEIGHBOUR-HOOD

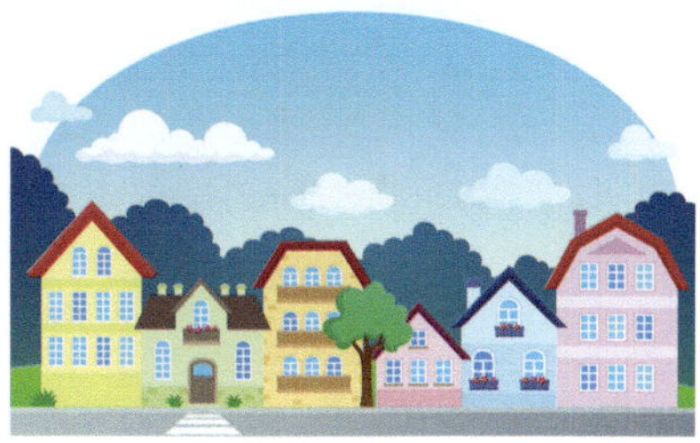

Figure 18.16.12

SIBLINGS

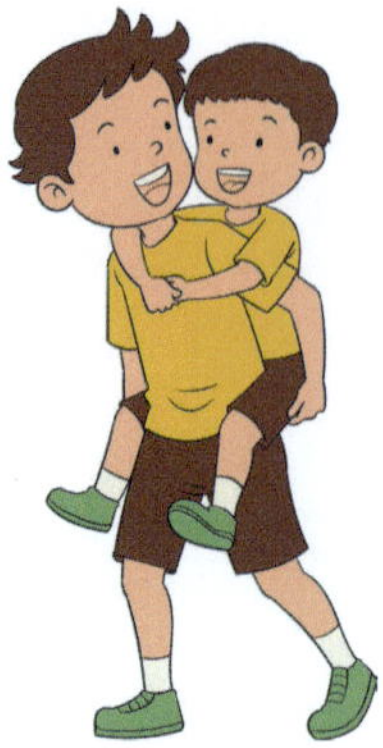

Figure 18.16.13

ROMANTIC PARTNER

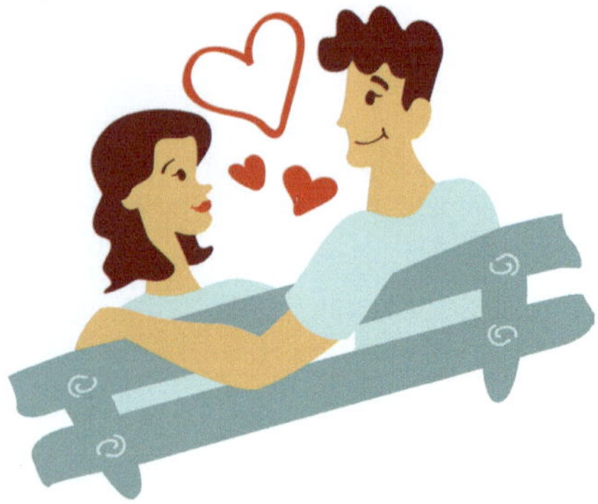

Figure 18.16.14

KNOWLEDGE

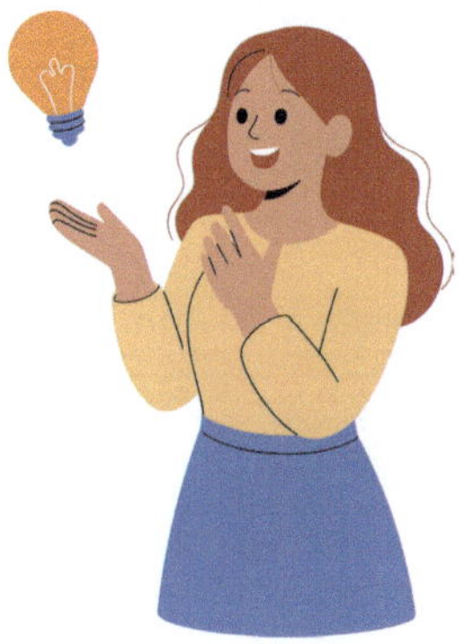

Figure 18.16.15

PERSONALITY

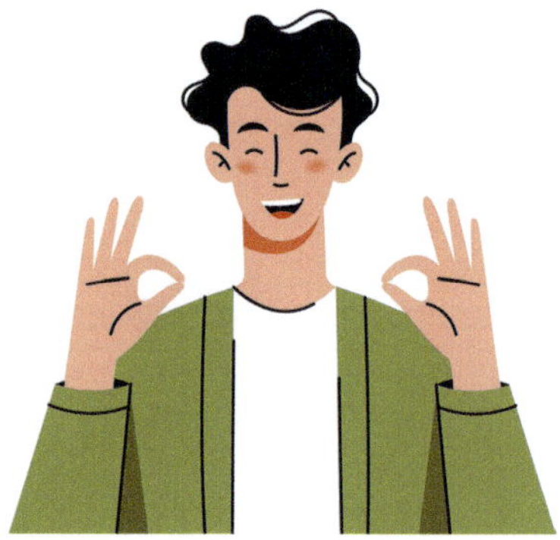

Figure 18.16.16

MENTAL HEALTH 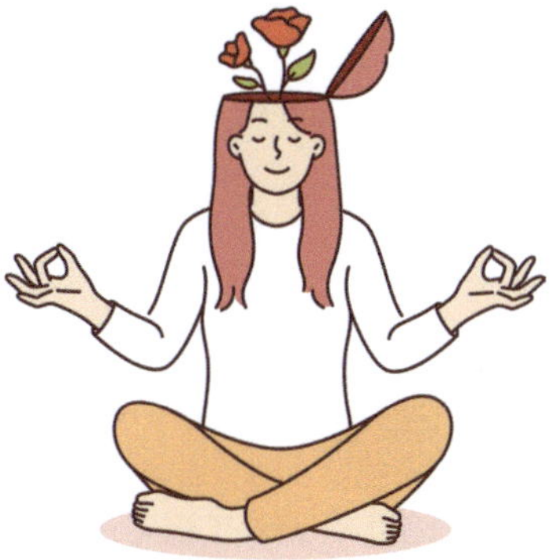 *Figure 18.16.17*	SELF-ESTEEM 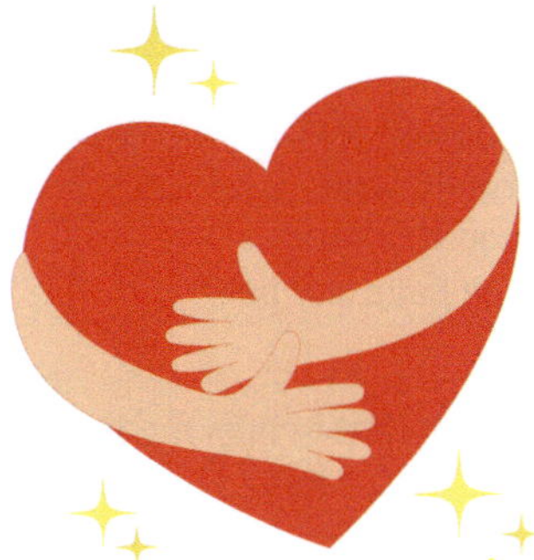 *Figure 18.16.18*

My Coat of Arms

Activity: In the **next page** you will see a coat of arms. **Each** of the **sections** has a **topic** for you to focus on. You can **fill them** in by **writing** or **drawing**. The sections are:

1. **A little about me:** Include your **name** and a little about yourself. For example:
   - Favouite food
   - Favourite colour
   - If you have any pets

2. **Something that brings me joy**: Think of **something or someone** that makes you feel **happy**. It does not have to be big or exciting, the 'little things in life' also count!

3. **Something I like about myself**: Think of something about **yourself** that makes you feel **happy** or **proud**. Think about your **personality**, **achievements**, **skills**...

4. **Something good in my world**: We have explored 'the world around us' in this session. Think of **something or someone** who is a **good influence** in **your life**. Why do they make your life better?

5. **Something I can overcome:** It would not be a coat of arms without winning a battle! Think of a **challenge** that you will face **in the group** (e.g. talking in public, making new friends...)? Then think about how you can **win** the battle against this **challenge**.

   ***Hint**: We are **stronger together**! Share your challenge with other members of the group. Maybe they have ideas on how you can win the battle, or even ideas on how they can help you!

My Coat of Arms

1.A little about me

2. Something I like about myself

3. Something that brings me joy

4. Something good in my world

5.Something I can overcome

Emotions Wheel

Telling Emotions Apart

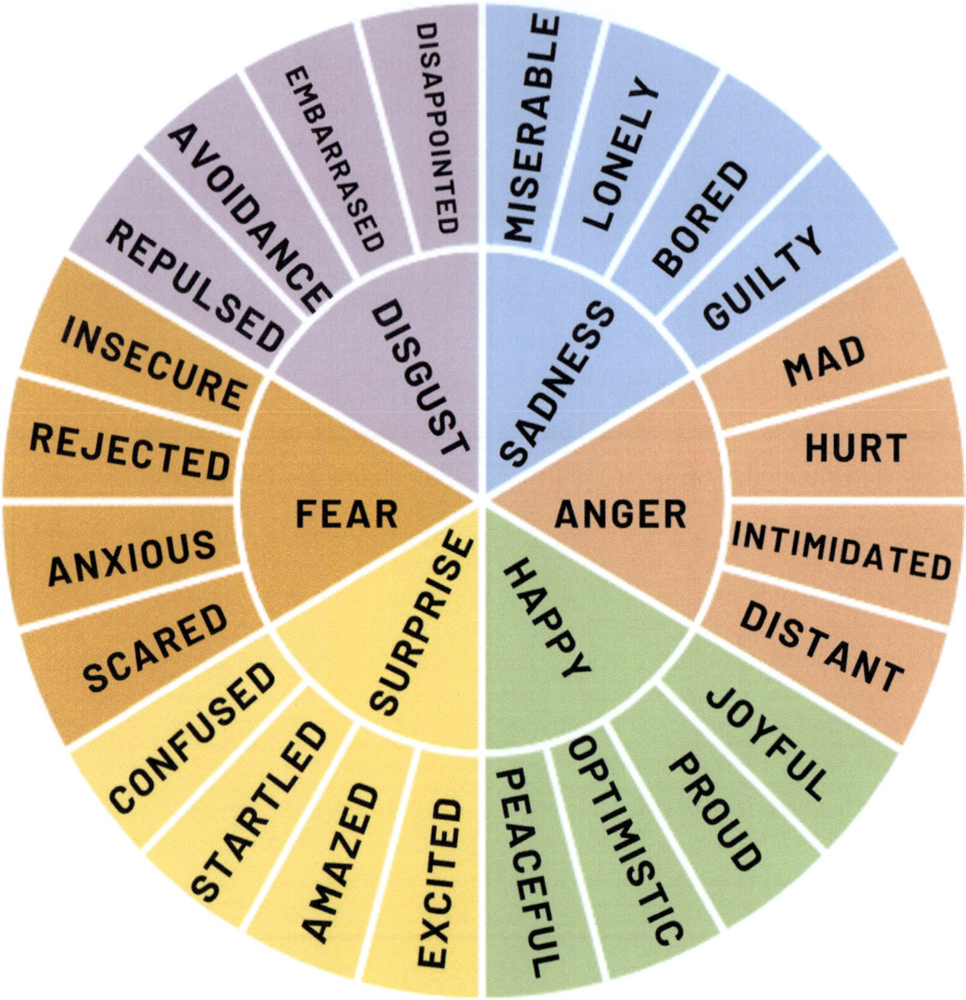

Figure 18.8

Physical Emotions in the Body Resource

'Physical Emotion in the Body' Visual Resource

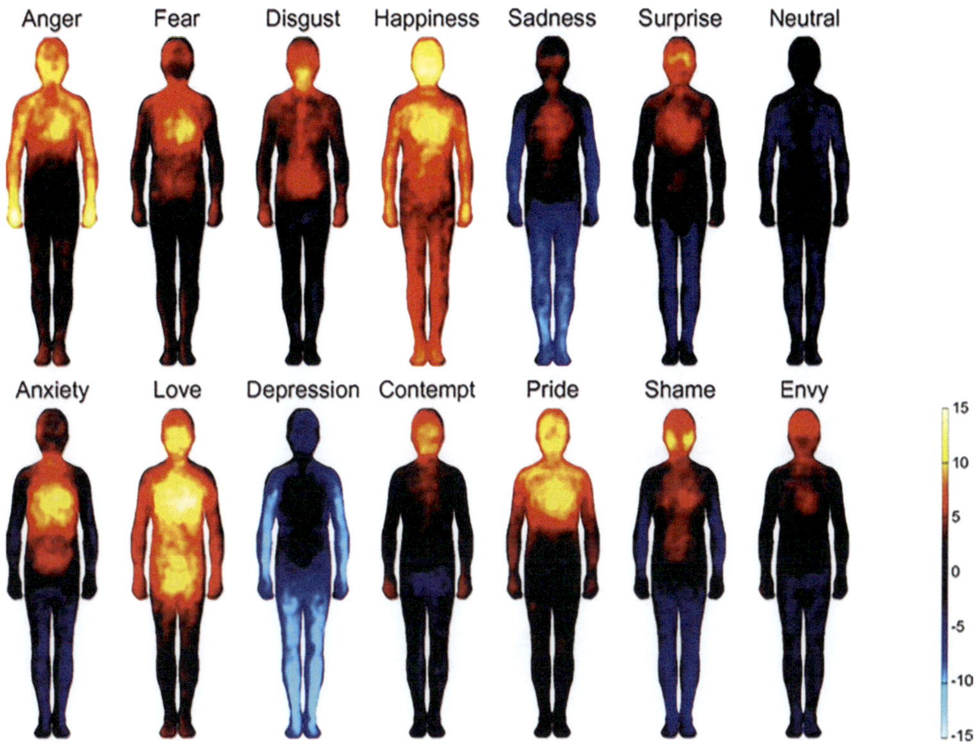

Figure 18.9 Visual body maps taken from a study of 'body maps' where people were asked to colour in the areas where they physically felt different emotions.

Source: Nummenmaa et al. (2014) – Permission provided by study authors[1].

Mapping Emotions Worksheet

Where does it feel?
Activity: Mapping emotions

- For each **song**, what **emotion** does it bring?
- Do the **emotions feel positive** or **negative?**
- How **intense** or **strong** do they feel?
- **Where** can you **feel them** in **your body**? Can you **label** the emotion?

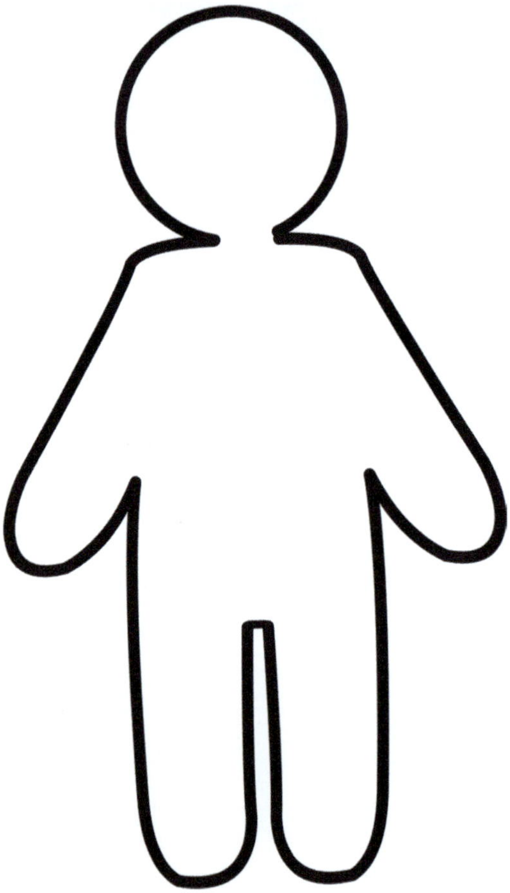

Figure 18.10

Positive or Negative?

There are **no 'good'** or **'bad' emotions**. But **some** do **feel nicer** than others.

Pleasant ⟷ Unpleasant

How Strong?

How intense does the **emotion feel**?

Can you feel the **same emotion** at **different levels**?

What changes at these times?

Think about your **physical feelings**, your **thoughts** and your **actions.**

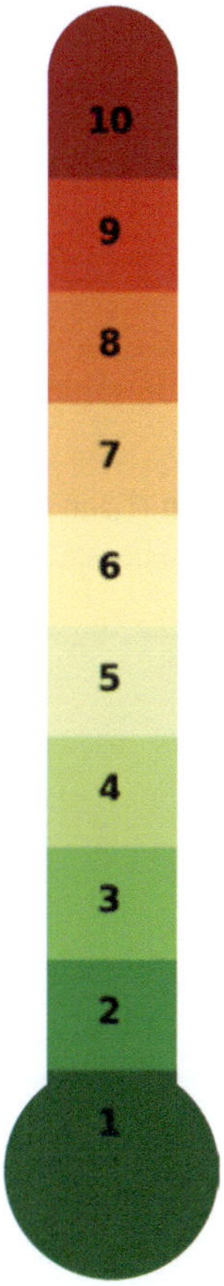

Figure 18.11

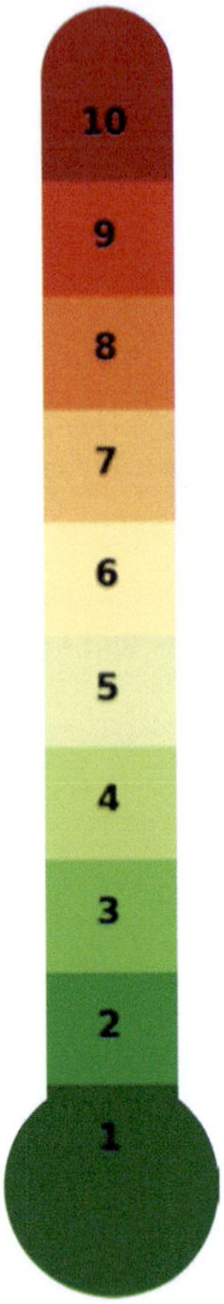

Figure 18.20.1

Emotion Thermometer Worksheet

Emotion Thermometer
This **Thermometer** shows the **'intensity'** (strength) of the **emotion** we are feeling.
10 is the **most intense** and **0** the **least intense.** You have already used a similar worksheet in Session 2 of SHERBET (when we did the music task!).

Emotion I will be **focusing** on:

Activity: Draw arrows to the **'intensity' levels** (numbers on the thermometer) that apply to the description.

After this point I feel **'out of control'**

After this point I feel **uncomfortable** and **struggle to manage** the emotion

Between these two points I can **manage the emotion** (I can feel the emotion without feeling too uncomfortable, overwhelmed or out of control)

Activity:
Are there any **situations** that make this **emotion** get very **intense**, very quickly? Give examples.

My 'Levels' of Emotion

Can you give some **'warning signs'** that **show other people** how **you are feeling**?
What are some **things you do** when the emotion is in this level of intensity?
What things might help you **'return to neutral'?**
What things would you **avoid** when you are trying to **'return to neutral'?**

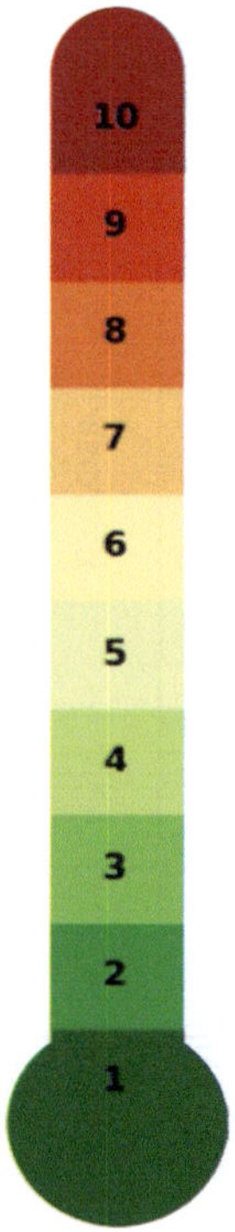

Out of Control			
Warning signs	**Things I might do**	**Helpful strategies**	**Unhelpful things**
Struggling to control			
Warning signs	**Things I might do**	**Helpful strategies**	**Unhelpful things**
Managing			
Warning signs	**Things I might do**	**Helpful strategies**	**Unhelpful things**

Figure 18.20.2

Emotion Thermometer Worksheet

Emotion Thermometer Prompts

The following can be printed and cut out to aid in the completion of the emotion thermometer activity.

Warning Signs

Feeling irritated	Headache	Heart beating faster
Feeling annoyed	Getting hot	Dizzy
Feeling uneasy	Sweating	Can't think straight
Feeling anxious	Shaking	Having angry thoughts
Feeling sad	Clenched jaw	Feel sick
Feeling energised	Thinking about hurting people	Feeling tense

Things I Do

Cry	Shout	Fight
Walk away	Scream	Break things
Shut down (stop talking/ listening)	Raising your voice	Punch things
Pacing	Doing something repetitive (like tapping)	Hurt people
Run away	Swearing	Hurt myself
Scowl or make an angry face	Say nasty things	Throw things

Strategies

Breathing exercises	Listen to music	Progressive muscle relaxation
Take a timeout	Recognise triggers	Count to 10
Challenge thoughts	Exercise	Walk away

Share how you are feeling	Use a fidget toy	Distraction techniques (such as 54321)
Stretch	Think about something else	Stop talking
Write down how you're feeling	Wait to respond	STOP technique
Do some sports	Go for a walk	Do some crafts
Punch something soft	Shake your hands/other parts of your body	Use a stress toy
Being with other people	Eating something nice	Picking an object and focusing on it very closely
Drawing, doodling or scribbling on paper	Allowing yourself to cry	Taking a shower
Having a warm drink	Looking up pictures of something you like	Calling a helpline, for example, Samaritans, Childline etc.
Writing a list of positive things in your life	Writing a list of goals for the future	Counting anything – patterns on wallpaper, bricks on a wall, ceiling tiles

Situations

Someone says something you find stupid	Someone says something you find rude	Someone talking when you are feeling tired
Being told off	Something breaking	Feeling like someone isn't listening
Feeling attacked	Losing at a game	Being talked over
Feeling alone	Things changing unexpectedly	Being ignored
Feeling put on the spot	Feeling confused	Loud people
Listening to music that annoys you	Something reminding you of a past experience	Loud noises

Deep Breathing Leaflet Trifold

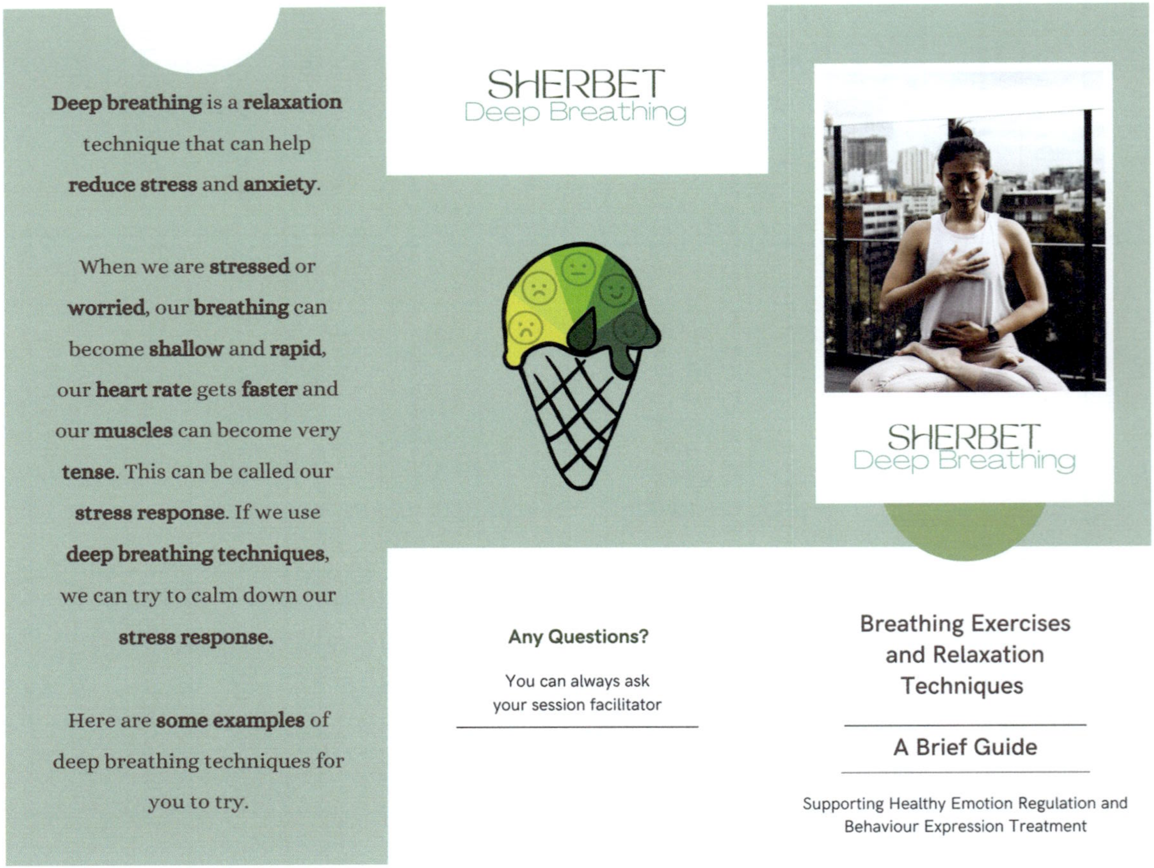
Deep breathing is a **relaxation** technique that can help **reduce stress** and **anxiety**.
When we are **stressed** or **worried**, our **breathing** can become **shallow** and **rapid**, our **heart rate** gets **faster** and our **muscles** can become very **tense**. This can be called our **stress response**. If we use **deep breathing techniques**, we can try to calm down our **stress response**.
Here are **some examples** of deep breathing techniques for you to try.
SHERBET
Deep Breathing
Any Questions?
You can always ask your session facilitator
SHERBET
Deep Breathing
Breathing Exercises and Relaxation Techniques
A Brief Guide
Supporting Healthy Emotion Regulation and Behaviour Expression Treatment

Figure 18.12

Belly Breathing

1. **Sit** or **lie** down
2. Place your **hands on** your **belly**
3. **Breathe** in through your **nose** (You will feel your **belly** get **bigger**)
4. Then, **breathe out** through your mouth (You will feel your **belly** go **smaller**)
5. Do this **5 times**.

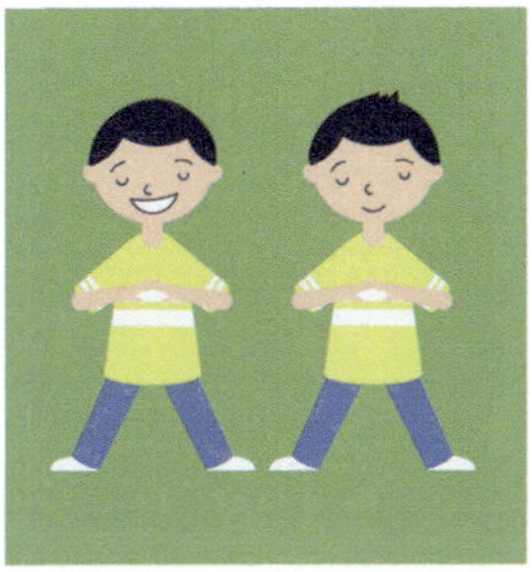

Star Breathing

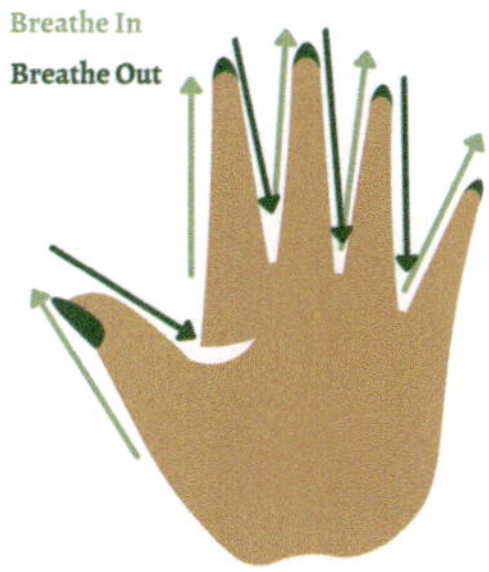

1. **Spread your hand** as if you were going to give someone a high five.
2. Use a finger on the other hand to **trace up** and **down** the fingers on your high five hand. (Do this **slowly**)
3. **Breathe in** as you **trace up** each finger
4. **Breathe out** when you **trace down** each finger

Muscle Relaxation

1. Take a **big breath in**
2. **Clench** your whole **body** (Squeeze your **fists, arms, stomach** and **legs**)
3. Keep squeezing for **10 seconds**
4. Slowly **breathe out** and **relax** your body
5. Do this **3 times.**

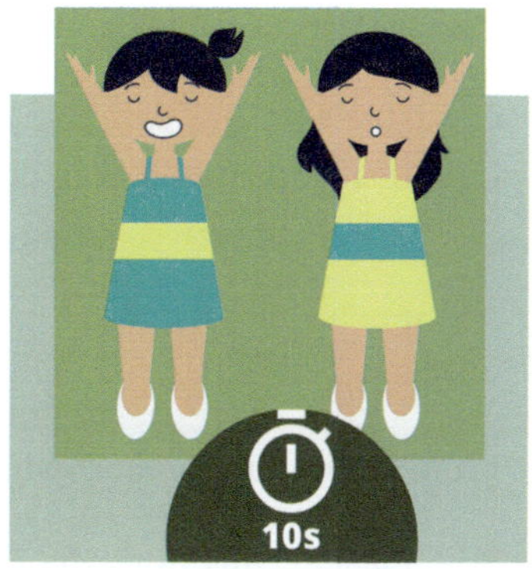

Figure 18.13

Character Scripts Resource 1

Recognising Emotions in Others – Scenarios for Session 4

Activity: These scenarios are to be used for Session 3 Task 3. Cut out the below scenarios and assign young people a scenario and role.

Scenario 1 – Laila

Child (Laila) and Parent (Nadia).

Laila is feeling really exhausted and doesn't want to go to school because she is bullied there – she hasn't told her mum about this. She is trying to convince mum to let her stay in bed.

(Emotions: exhaustion, fear, dread)

Scenario 1 – Nadia

Child (Laila) and Parent (Nadia).

Nadia wants Laila to get up and go to school. Laila has been doing this a lot recently which has been making Nadia late for work. Nadia is worried that she will be fired if she keeps arriving late, her benefits wouldn't be enough to support the family. She also wants Laila to go to school so she can be well educated and have a better future.

(Emotions: frustration, worry, hope)

Scenario 2 – Jessie

Sam and Jessie are friends who are hanging out together.

Jessie has recently broken up with a partner and was looking forward to meeting up with Sam to talk to a friend about it. Sam keeps looking at their phone and doesn't seem to be listening. Jessie continues to try to talk to Sam, but gets more and more wound up as this goes on.

(Emotions: sad, disappointed, angry)

Scenario 2 – Sam

Sam and Jessie are friends who are hanging out together.

Sam is waiting for results to a test they had at the doctor's. They don't want to tell Jessie about this, as they feel embarrassed about the problem. If they miss the phone call from the doctor, they've been told they won't be able to speak to the doctor for another week. Sam keeps looking at their phone to make sure they don't miss the call. Sam is struggling to listen to what Jessie is saying.

(Emotions: anxious, nervous, embarrassed)

Scenario 3 – Ms Collins

Ms Collins is usually a patient teacher; however, she has had a bad day today. She received a huge vet bill for her dog this before work and is worried about how she will pay it. She then blew a tire on the way to work but was told she needed to come into work as there was no one else to teach her classes. She's been feeling like everything is building up inside of her all day, so when Fidel walks in late, she's had enough. She tells Fidel off in front of everyone and this turns into a big argument.

(Emotions: stressed, anxious, frustrated)

Scenario 3 – Fidel

Fidel is a pupil in Ms Collins' class.

Fidel is usually chill; however, he has had a bad day today… He had an argument with his carer this morning and then one of his friends was 'taking the micky' out of his hair at lunch. He comes into class late as he's been trying to calm himself down in the toilet. He walks straight to his desk and doesn't say anything as he's trying to stay calm. Ms Collins tells him off for being late and they end up in an argument.

(Emotions: rejected, hurt, threatened, angry)

Social Story Worksheet

What do you mean?

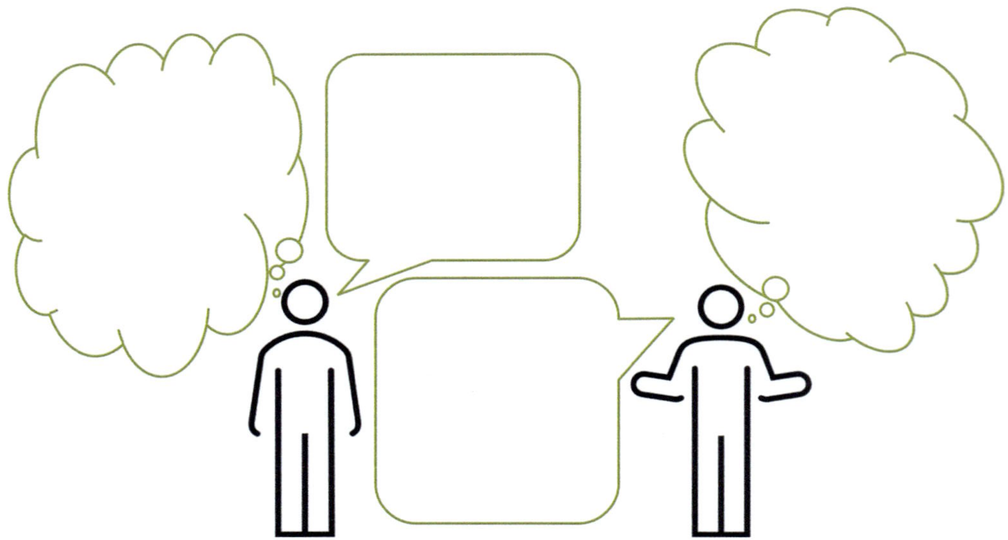

Figure 18.14

Cognitive Biases Worksheet

Thinking Errors

Cognitive biases (a.k.a. **'thinking errors', 'mental mistakes'**) are errors in our thinking that we make **without even knowing** we have **made them** (unconsciously).

Thinking errors can make us **see** the **world** in a **less rational** or **accurate way.**

These are **automatic processes** which we developed to **make quicker decisions**. However, they can also be **unhelpful.**

Activity

- Here are some **examples** of **thinking errors** that you might have seen or experienced.
- **As a group** we will think of times where we have **seen these thinking errors** in action.
- **Write** down **one example** for each thinking error.

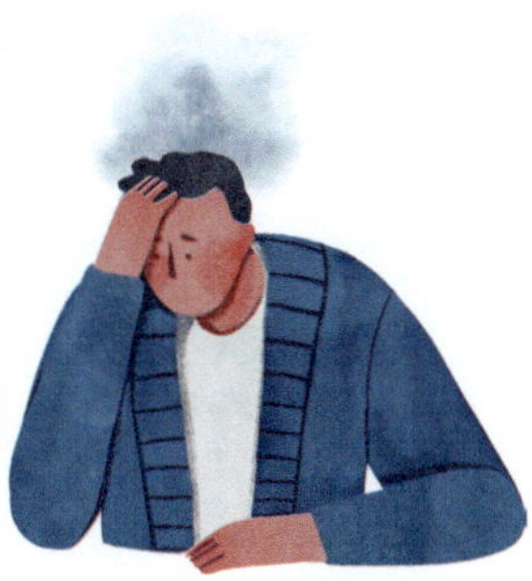 *Figure 18.26.1*	**Rumination or 'Sticky Thoughts'** This is a state where we may **get 'stuck'** in specific thoughts. Overthinking can lead to the emotion getting more intense.	
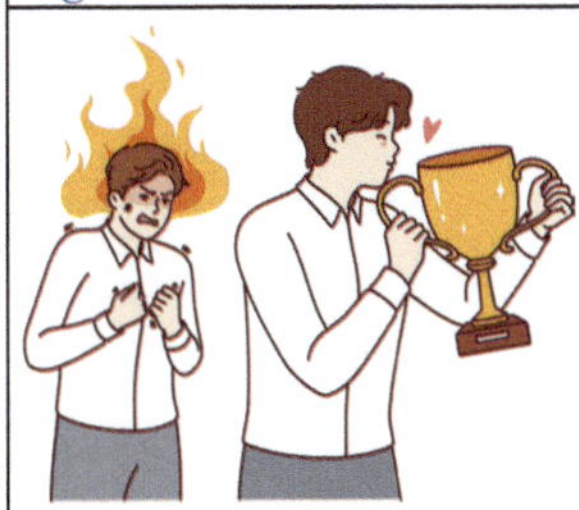 *Figure 18.26.2*	**All or nothing thinking** **Extremes** in our thinking. These can refer to yourself or to other people. For example – 'If I'm not perfect, I have failed', 'Either I do it right or not at all'.	
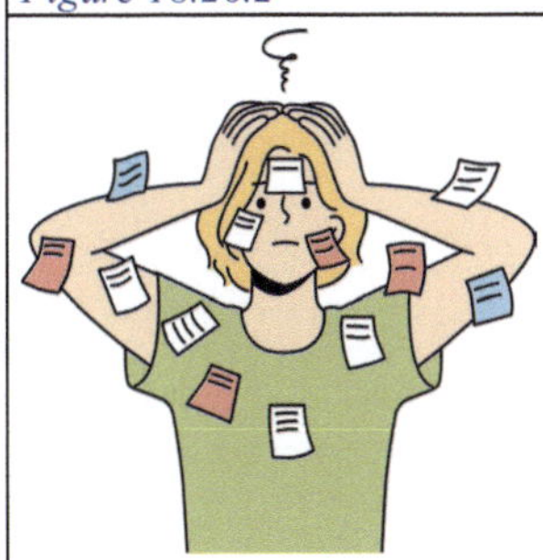 *Figure 18.26.3*	**Over generalising** Seeing a **pattern** in a **single event**, making **generalised conclusions.** Some common words associated with this are: never, always, nothing, everything... For example, 'Everything is always rubbish'.	

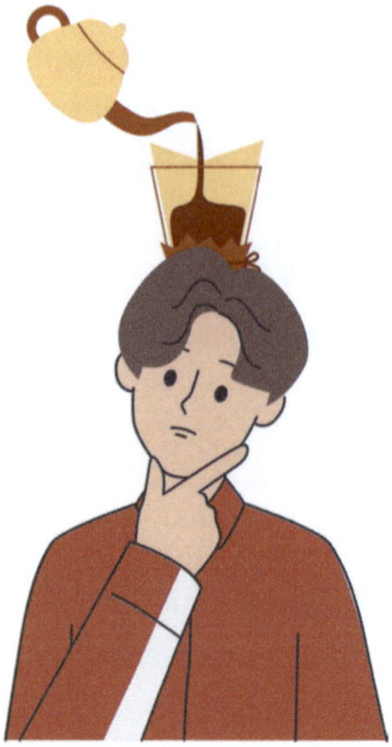 *Figure 18.26.4*	**Mental filter** **Paying attention** only to **certain information**.	
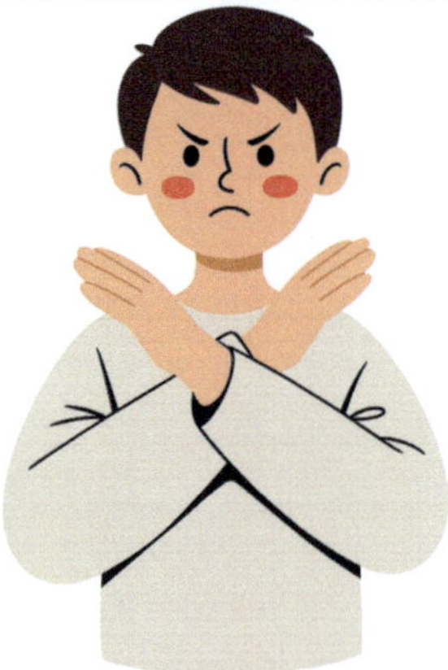 *Figure 18.26.5*	**Disqualifying the positive** Saying that when something **positive** happens 'it **doesn't count'**.	
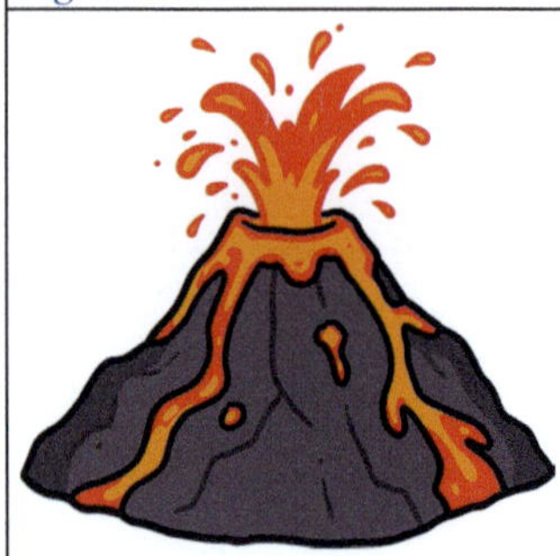 *Figure 18.26.6*	**Magnification** Blowing things **out of proportion.** Making a **situation bigger** than it really is.	

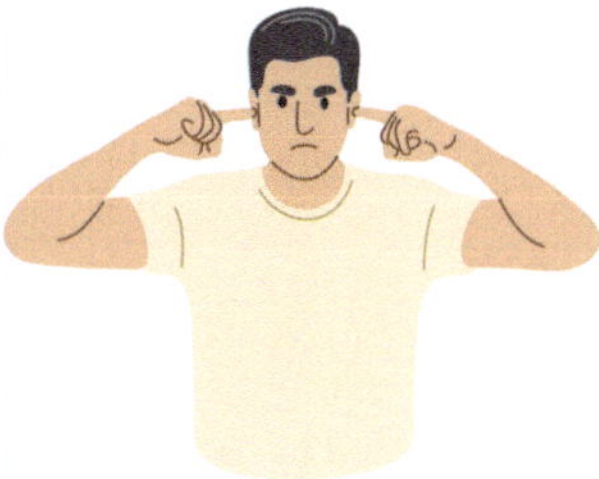 *Figure 18.26.7*	**Minimisation** 'Shrinking' something to make it **seem less important**.	
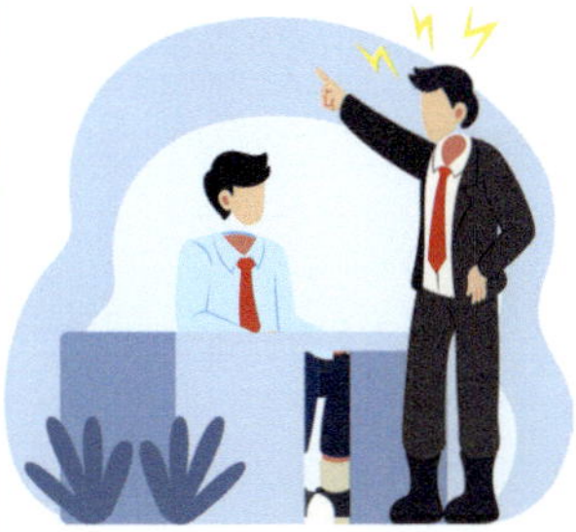 *Figure 18.26.8*	**Critical words** Using **critical words** like 'should', 'must', or 'ought' can make us **feel guilty**, or like we have **already failed**. This is also true when we say them to other people – they will likely feel frustrated.	
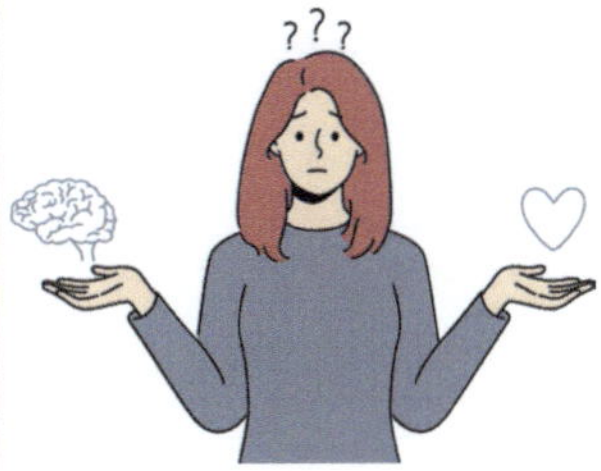 *Figure 18.26.9*	**Emotional reasoning** Assuming that because we **feel a certain way**, what we think **must be true**.	
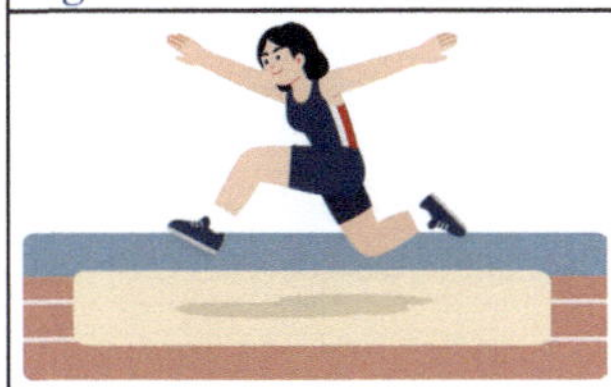 *Figure 18.26.10*	**Jumping to conclusions** Can include: - **'Mind reading'** (imagining that we know what others are thinking). - **'Fortune telling'** (imagining that we know what is going to happen).	

CBT Model Worksheet

The 'Hot Cross Bun'

Activity 1

Our emotions, sensations, thoughts and behaviours are all connected. We can get 'stuck' in a loop that keeps a problem going. Consider your main challenge that you wanted to focus on (e.g. hitting others, avoiding things, getting excluded…). What emotions, sensations, thoughts and behaviours are part of this loop?

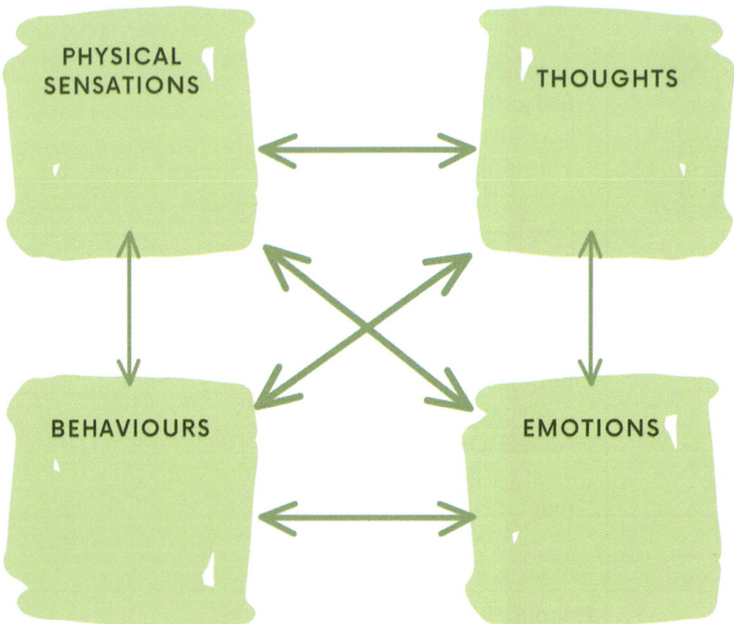

Figure 18.15

Activity 2

What parts of the hot cross bun do you have more control over? Where can you start to make a change?
What changes could you make? For example, more helpful thoughts or behaviours that can help you break the loop.

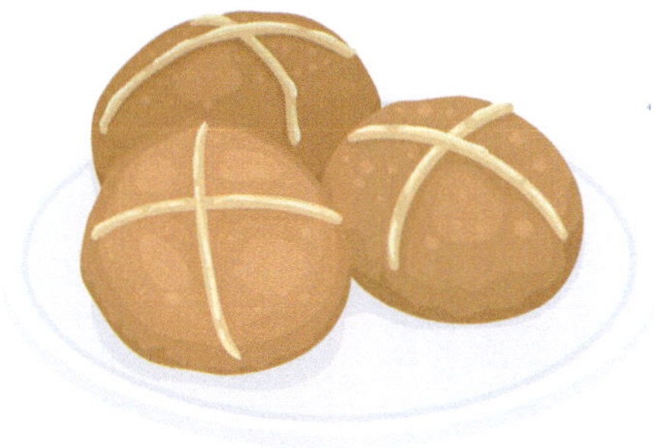

Figure 18.16

Thought Diary Worksheet

Thought Diary

Thought diaries can help us **look back** on **what happened** in our day and **challenge** how we **responded** in **difficult situations.**

They are a helpful tool to help us **understand** how our **thoughts, feelings** and **behaviours** all link together.

Reviewing situations like this can help us spot any **patterns** in how we **respond** to **difficult things**, but also **celebrate** if we **act positively** in a difficult situation.

Activity

- **Complete** the **thought diary** throughout the week. There are some **options** on **when** to **use the diary**:
    - At the **end** of the **day**: This may be **useful if** you still **struggle to stop and think** when you are in a difficult situation, or if you **struggle to find time** in the day to stop and think. At the end of the day, you can **choose one important moment** or difficult situation and **think about it** when writing the diary.
    - When you are **in** a **difficult situation**: This may be **useful** to **practice stopping and thinking** before acting. If you **realise** you are **in** a **difficult situation** (e.g. angry at someone, anxious about something…) try to **take a break** from the situation, **go** to a **quiet place,** and **fill in** this **thought diary**. This may help you **decide what to do**, so you can **act** in a way that is **kinder** and more **helpful** for your goals.
- Use the columns to fill in **what happened**, your **thoughts, emotions, physical feelings** and **behaviours.**
- Use the **last column** to **reflect** on if you could have **responded differently.**

Date	*What happened?* *- Describe the situation* *-Where were you?* *- Who were you with?*	*Thoughts* *-Unhelpful thoughts* *-Helpful thoughts*	*Emotions* *-What were they?* *- Intensity?* *0-10*	*Physical feelings* *- For example, stomach ache/ heart beating quickly*	*Behaviour* *-What did you do?*	*Could I have thought or done something differently?* *-Any thinking errors?* *- What will I change for next time?* *- What helped that I can use again?*

Character Scripts Resource 2

Communication Styles – Session 7 Prompts

Continuing from Session 4 Scenarios

Scenario 1

Daughter (Laila) and mother (Nadia).

Laila is feeling really exhausted and doesn't want to go to school because she is bullied there – she hasn't told her mum about this. She is trying to convince mum to let her stay in bed.

(Emotions: exhaustion, fear, dread)

Nadia wants Laila to get up and go to school. Laila has been doing this a lot recently which has been making Nadia late for work. Nadia is worried that she will be fired if she keeps arriving late, her benefits wouldn't be enough to support the family. She also wants Laila to go to school so she can be well educated and have a better future.

(Emotions: frustration, worry, hope)

<u>Question to ask group:</u> How do you think Nadia could approach Laila in this situation?

<u>Examples of what Nadia might say:</u>

Passive: Ok well I guess if you don't want to go I'll leave you alone.

Aggressive: You are such a spoilt brat! I need to go to work to pay the bills and look after this family. You've got a great opportunity to better yourself and you don't appreciate it.

Assertive: Laila, I can see you really don't want to go to school but sometimes we have to do the things we don't want to do. This seems to be happening a lot recently, is there anything you need to talk about? Maybe we can work together to find a solution.

Scenario 2

Sam and Jessie are friends who are hanging out together.

Sam is waiting for results to a test they had at the doctor's. They don't want to tell Jessie about this, as they feel embarrassed about the problem. If they miss the phone call from the doctor, they've been told they won't be able to speak to the doctor for another week. Sam keeps looking at their phone to make sure they don't miss the call. Sam is struggling to listen to what Jessie is saying.

(Emotions: anxious, nervous, embarrassed)

Jessie has recently broken up with a partner and was looking forward to meeting up with Sam to talk to a friend about it. Sam keeps looking at their phone and doesn't seem to be listening. Jessie continues to try to talk to Sam, but gets more and more wound up as this goes on.

(Emotions: sad, disappointed, angry)

Question to ask group: How do you think Sam could approach Jessie about this situation?

Examples of what Jessie might say:

Passive: Well, I guess I'll just go home then.

Aggressive: You are so rude. How dare you treat me like this?! I'm meant to be your friend.

Assertive: I was really looking forward to seeing you today but you seem distracted, this is making me feel ignored and alone. Is there something bothering you?

Scenario 3

Fidel is a pupil in Ms Collins' class.

Fidel is usually chill; however, he has had a bad day today... He had an argument with his carer this morning and then one of his friends was 'taking the micky' out of his hair at lunch. He comes into class late as he's been trying to calm himself down in the toilet. He walks straight to his desk and doesn't say anything as he's trying to stay calm. Ms Collins tells him off for being late and they end up in an argument.

(Emotions: rejected, hurt, threatened, angry)

Ms Collins is usually a patient teacher; however, she has had a bad day today. She received a huge vet bill for her dog this morning before work and is worried about how she will pay it. She then crashed her car on the way to work but was told she needed to come into work as there was no one else to teach her classes. She's been feeling like everything is building up inside of her all day, so when Fidel walks in late, she's had enough. She tells Fidel off in front of everyone and this turns into a big argument.

(Emotions: stressed, anxious, frustrated)

Question to ask group: In this situation Ms Collins tells Fidel off for being late. What communication style do you think she could have used for this? What might have been better?

Examples of what Ms Collins Might Say:

Passive: *says nothing*

Aggressive: What time do you call this? One rule for you and another for everyone else, is it?!

Assertive: Fidel, I have to remind you that being on time is a school expectation. Maybe we can talk about the reason for this after class.

Question to ask group: Fidel doesn't like being told off so responds aggressively, how else do you think Fidel could respond better?

Examples of what Fidel Might Say:

Passive: Whatever.

Aggressive: You stupid cow. You don't even know what I've been through today. Shut your mouth.

Assertive: Ms Collins, I'm sorry for being late. But there was a reason for this. I can explain after class.

New Scenarios for Session 7

Attendees may model the general situations described below. Some examples of possible responses have been provided.

You want to ask someone to stop doing something irritating
Passive: That noise is a bit annoying.
Aggressive: Will you pack it in before I knock you out?
Assertive: Certain noises can make me feel uncomfortable. Could you stop doing that whilst I'm here, please?

Someone asks you to share your food – you don't want to
Passive: Yeah, sure, have some.
Aggressive: No way, get lost!
Assertive: No, sorry. It's all I have for today and I'm still hungry. I know you get it.

Someone you don't particularly like very much asks you to go to the cinema
Passive: Erm, I'm not sure. Maybe.
Aggressive: Hahaha as if!
Assertive: That's a really kind offer but I'd rather not, thank you.

You disagree with what someone else is saying
Passive: Yeah, you're probably right.
Aggressive: You're an idiot why would you even think that?
Assertive: I get why you might think that but I don't agree.

Greeting Game

The facilitator should ask the young people to split into A's and B's.
B's will be instructed to go outside the room. They will be given a scenario to keep to themselves. B's will then return to the room, and one at a time and greet their partner (A's). Partners should try to guess B's relationship/feelings towards them. This can also be opened up to the group for discussion.

Scenarios:
Greeting the queen
Greeting your favourite celebrity
Greeting your friend
Greeting your boss
Greeting a teacher

Greeting your enemy

Following the activity facilitators should encourage discussion to reflect on this activity such as:

- What was different in each situation?
- Who are the people they communicate with? Are there differences in how they interact with these people?
- What would happen if you greeted your friends in the same way you greeted someone in authority? And vice versa.

Conversation points:

- Knowing how to communicate with people in the right context for a given situation is an important skill, as there are often unspoken rules and standards that are expected.
- For example, it's common practice in the professional world to shake hands with people when meeting, rather than offering a high-five or a hug.
- We might use slang with our friends when talking about what happened at school or at a party, but we would usually use different words and mannerisms when telling our parents, the same information.

Reviewing Achievements

Remember Your Strengths

Write answers to these prompts:

The most **important things** that I have **learned** in **SHERBET**:

Something I have **learned** or realised in **SHERBET** that I **do not** want to **forget**:

For example, coping skills, something helpful/unhelpful I do...

Something I **did well/achieved** in SHERBET:

Remember the things you have achieved so far!

Keep working towards your goals – you can do it!

SHERBET

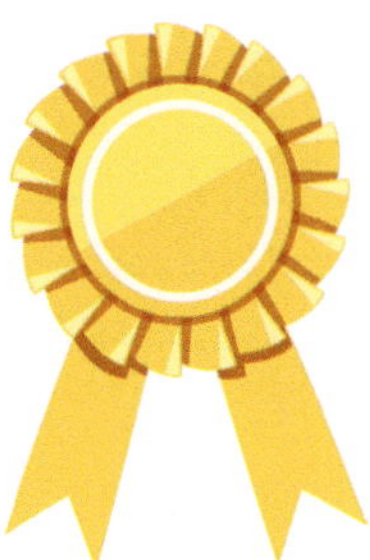

Figure 18.17

Reference

1 Nummenmaa, L., Glerean, E., Hari, R., & Hietanen, J. K. (2014). Bodily maps of emotions. *Proceedings of the National Academy of Sciences*, *111*(2), 646–651.

19 Summary Workbook

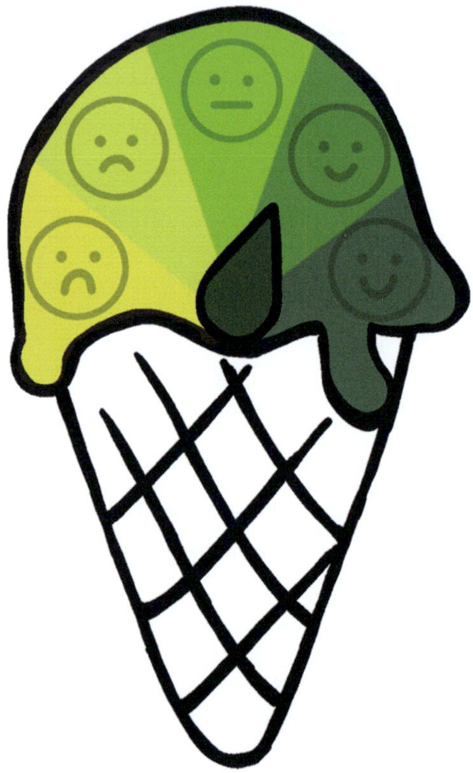

Figure 19.1

DOI: 10.4324/9781003666738-19

SHERBET

Supporting Healthy Emotion Regulation and Behavioural Expression Treatment
COMPLETER'S WORKBOOK
Name:

Steps for Change

NAME:

Steps for Change

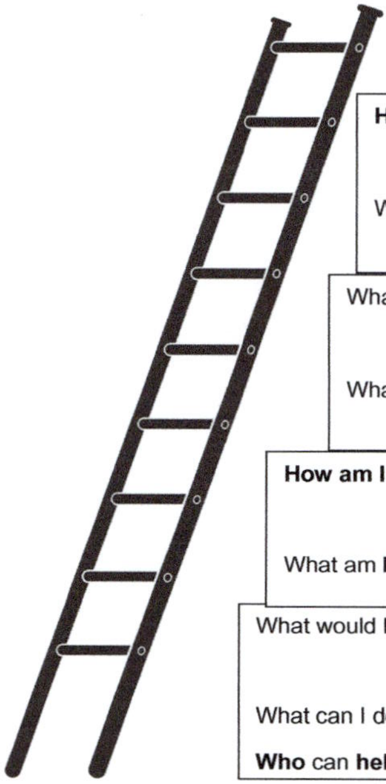

My Goal:

What **good things** will I get **from achieving my goal?**

How do I know I **achieved** my Goal?

What things may I **learn** in the program that can **help me achieve** my goal?

What do **I want** to **achieve** in this first step?

What things do **I need** to **do** to achieve it?

How am I now? Where am I in relation to my goal?

What am **I doing about it now**?

What would **happen** if I got **worse**?

What can I do if **I struggle** to achieve my goal?

Who can **help** me?

The World Around Us

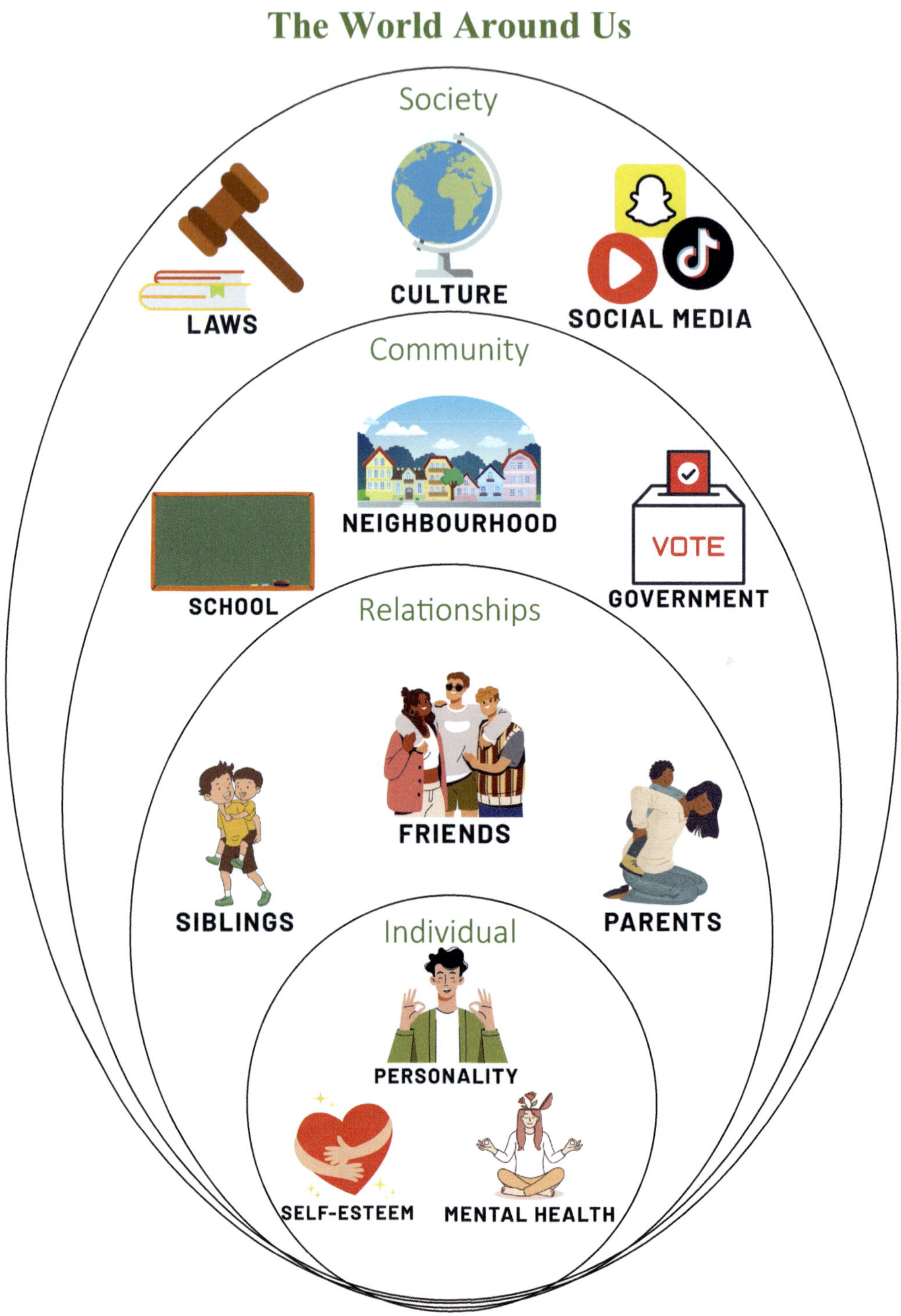

Influencing Life

We need to **focus** our **energies** on what we **can control** and **influence!**

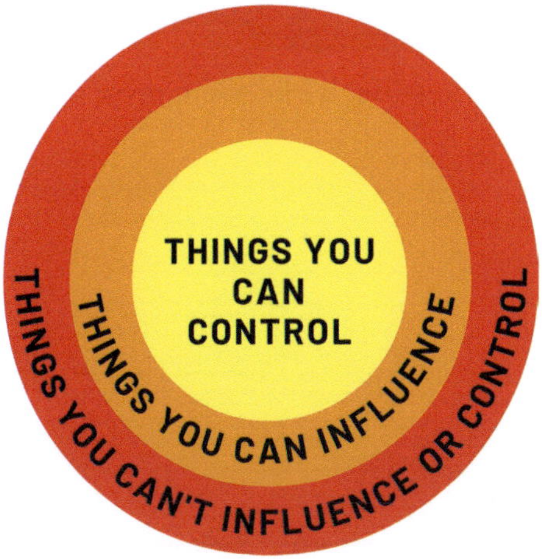

Figure 19.2

1. CIRCLE OF **CONTROL:** What we can **directly control**
2. CIRCLE OF **INFLUENCE:** The **worries** that we **can do something about**
3. CIRCLE OF **CONCERN:** Wide range of **worries** which **we cannot change** right now

My Coat of Arms

Activity: In the **next page** you will see a coat of arms. **Each** of the **sections** has a **topic** for you to focus on. You can **fill them** in by **writing** or **drawing**. The sections are:

1. A little about me: Include your name and a little about yourself. For example:
   - Favouite food
   - Favourite colour
   - If you have any pets
2. Something that brings me joy: Think of something or someone that makes you feel happy. It does not have to be big or exciting, the 'little things in life' also count!
3. Something I like about myself: Think of something about yourself that makes you feel happy or proud. Think about your personality, achievements, skills...
4. Something good in my world: We have explored 'the world around us' in this session. Think of something or someone who is a good influence in your life. Why do they make your life better?
5. Something I can overcome: It would not be a coat of arms without winning a battle! Think of a challenge that you will face in the group (e.g. talking in public, making new friends...)? Then think about how you can win the battle against this challenge.

*Hint: We are stronger together! Share your challenge with other members of the group. Maybe they have ideas on how you can win the battle, or even ideas on how they can help you!

My Coat of Arms

1.A little about me

2. Something I like about myself

3. Something that brings me joy

4. Something good in my world

5.Something I can overcome

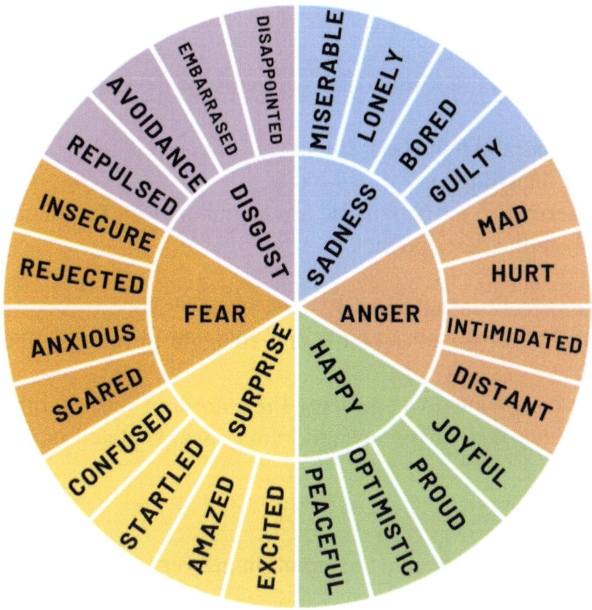

Figure 19.3

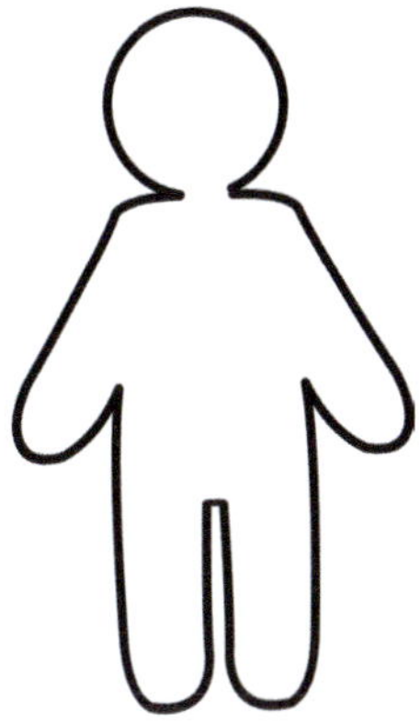

Figure 19.4

Where Does It Feel?

Activity: Mapping emotions. We can feel emotions in our bodies. For example, clenching our fists, butterflies in our tummies. Recognising these signs can help us recognise the emotion and act early on it!

There are **no 'good'** or **'bad' emotions**. But **some** do **feel nicer** than others.

Remember that all emotions have some positive and negative functions. The important bit is how we react to the emotion.

For example, anxiety can help us avoid dangerous things and keep ourselves safe. However, if anxiety gets too strong, we might avoid safe things that we like because we find them too scary. Then anxiety looks like a problem because it stops us from doing things we value – but really the emotion is not the problem, it's how we react to it!

Emotion Thermometer

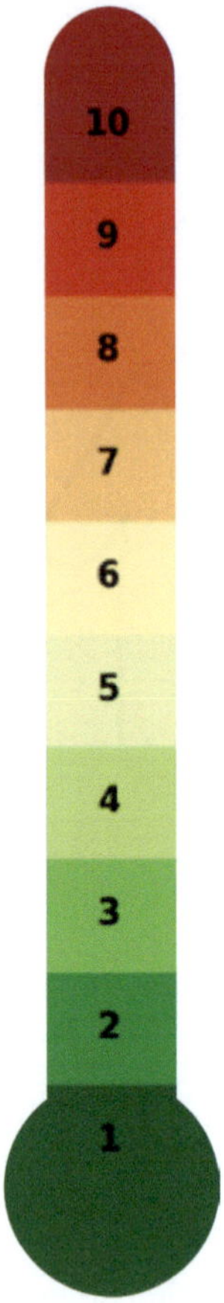

This **thermometer** shows the **'intensity'** (strength) of the **emotion** we are feeling.
10 is the **most intense** and **0** the **least intense.**
Emotion I will be **focusing** on:
Activity: Draw arrows to the **'intensity' levels** (numbers on the thermometer) that apply to the description.

After this point I feel **'out of control'**
After this point I feel **uncomfortable** and **struggle to manage** the emotion
Between these two points I can **manage the emotion** (I can feel the emotion without feeling too uncomfortable, overwhelmed or out of control)

Activity:
Are there any **situations** that make this **emotion** get very **intense**, very quickly? Give examples.

My ‘Levels’ of Emotion

Can you give some **‘warning signs’** that **show other people** how **you are feeling**?
What are some **things you do** when the emotion is in this level of intensity?
What things might help you **‘return to neutral’?**
What things would you **avoid** when you are trying to **‘return to neutral’?**

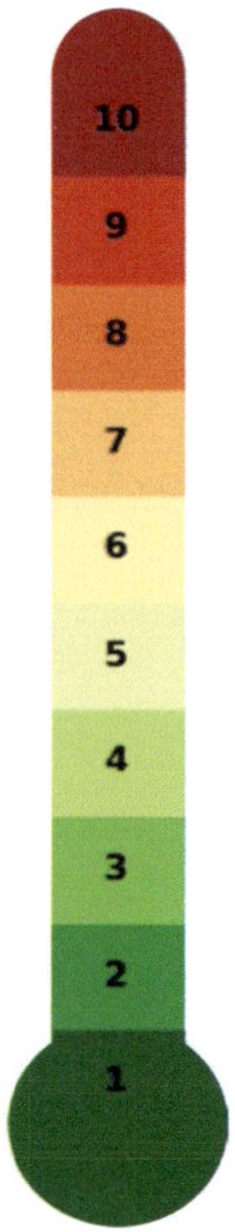

Out of Control			
Warning signs	**Things I might do**	**Helpful strategies**	**Unhelpful things**
Struggling to control			
Warning signs	**Things I might do**	**Helpful strategies**	**Unhelpful things**
Managing			
Warning signs	**Things I might do**	**Helpful strategies**	**Unhelpful things**

Thinking Errors

Cognitive biases (a.k.a. 'thinking errors', 'mental mistakes') are errors in our thinking that we make without even knowing we have made them (unconsiously).
Thinking errors can make us see the world in a less rational or accurate way.
These are automatic processes which we developed to make quicker decisions. However, they can also be unhelpful.

Activity

- Here are some **examples** of **thinking errors** that you might have seen or experienced.
- **As a group** we will think of times where we have **seen these thinking errors** in action.
- **Write** down **one example** for each thinking error.

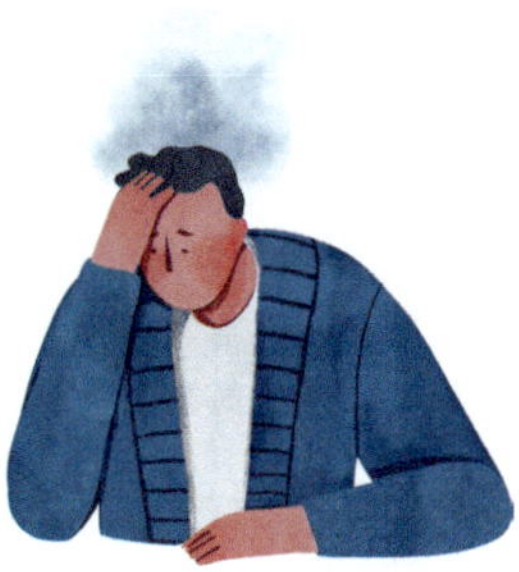 *Figure 18.26.1*	Rumination or 'Sticky Thoughts' This is a state where we may get 'stuck' in specific thoughts. Overthinking can lead to the emotion getting more intense.	After a fight thinking about it a lot keeps me angry.
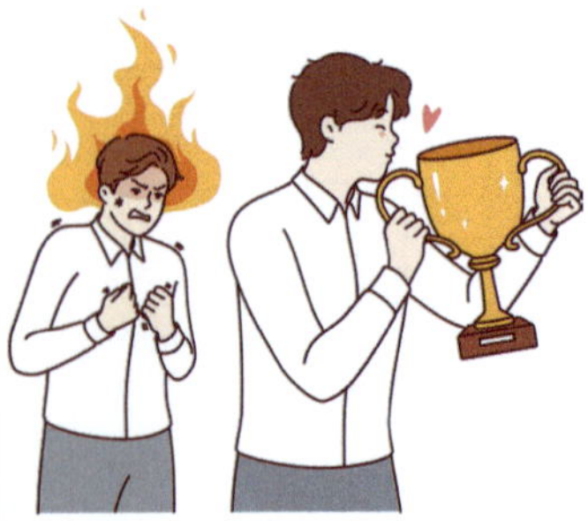 *Figure 18.26.2*	All or nothing thinking Extremes in our thinking. These can refer to yourself or to other people. For example, 'if I'm not perfect, I have failed', 'either I do it right or not at all'.	Either I do it right or not at all. I'm not going to get an 8 in my exams so what is the point in trying?

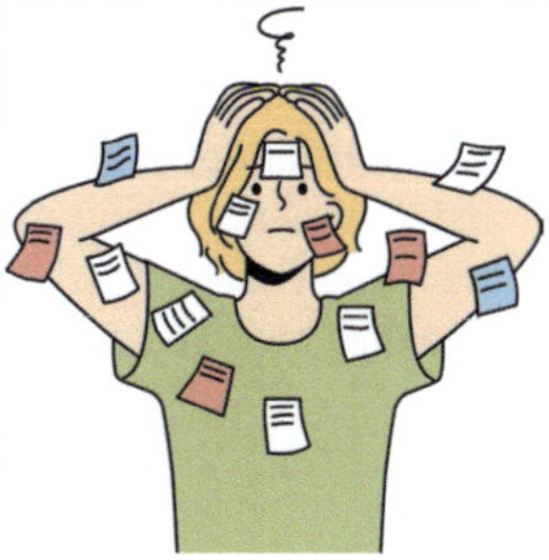 *Figure 18.26.3*	Over generalising Seeing a pattern in a single event, making generalised conclusions. Some common words associated with this are: never, always, nothing, everything... For example, 'everything is always rubbish'.	I had one argument with a friend and they stopped talking to me. I am a horrible friend and will never make friends again.
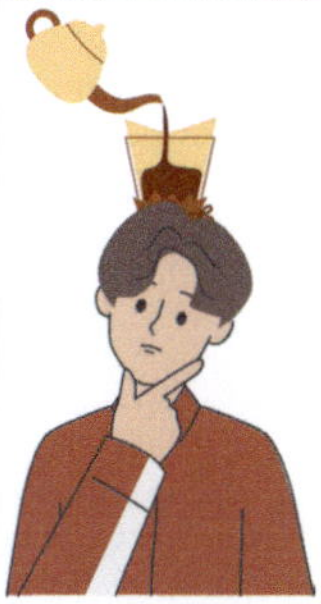 *Figure 18.26.4*	Mental filter Paying attention only to certain information.	Some people say good things about me and say they believe in me. I often forget that they have said this. I always remember when people have said bad things about me.
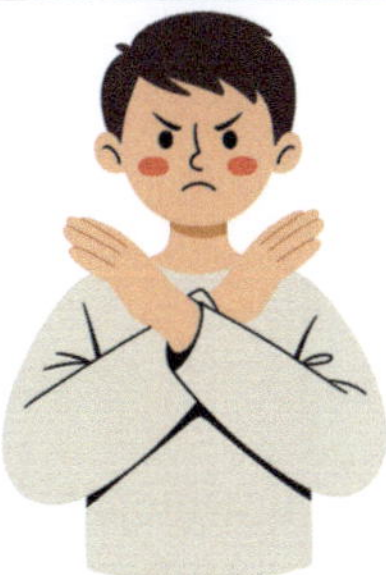 *Figure 18.26.5*	Disqualifying the positive saying that when something positive happens 'it doesn't count'.	I know I managed to explain myself and stay calm this time but I still don't think that is a skill I have. This time must have been a coincidence, it's still not in my control.
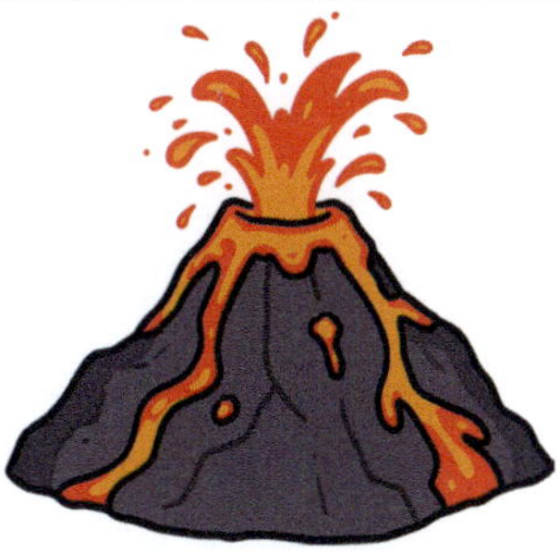 *Figure 18.26.6*	Magnification Blowing things out of proportion. Making a **situation bigger** than it really is.	I get beaten at a videogame online. I get incredibly angry and shout nasty things at the person and smash my controller.

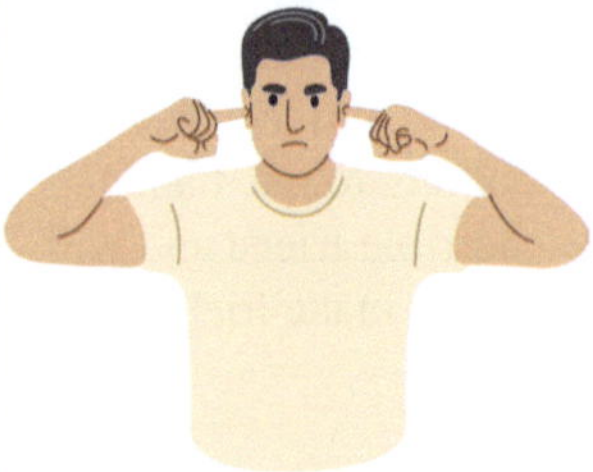 *Figure 18.26.7*	Minimisation 'Shrinking' something to make it seem less important.	I broke my friend's phone but they had it coming for not listening to me and they're my friend so they won't care. If they care they are 'weak'.
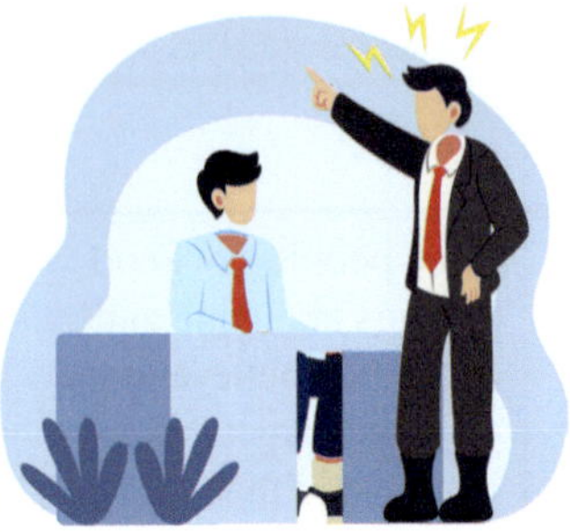 *Figure 18.26.8*	Critical words Using critical words like 'should', 'must', or 'ought' can make us feel guilty, or like we have already failed. This is also true when we say them to other people – they will likely feel frustrated.	You are **always** so disrespectful, you **should** get your act together. You **never** care about others.
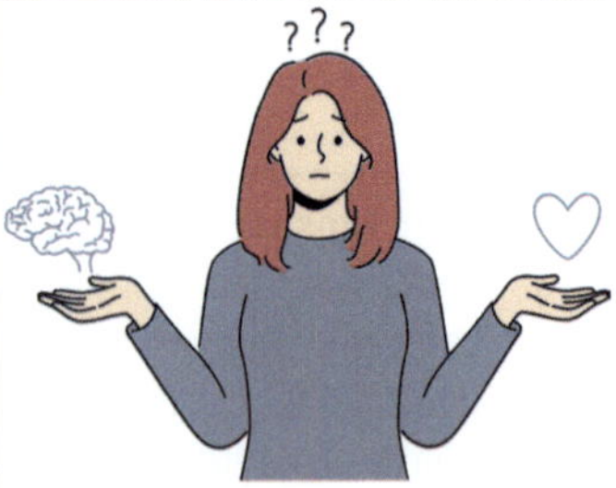 *Figure 18.26.9*	Emotional reasoning Assuming that because we feel a certain way, what we think must be true.	I feel really guilty and embarrassed so others must think that I am embarrassing.
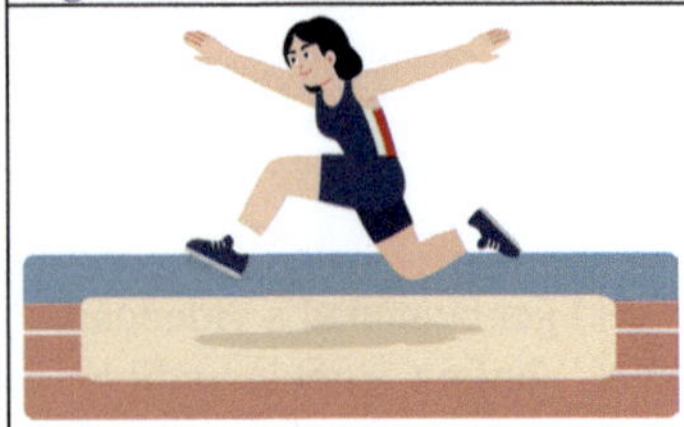 *Figure 18.26.10*	Jumping to conclusions can include: - 'Mind reading' (imagining that we know what others are thinking). - 'Fortune telling' (imagining that we know what is going to happen).	'This person is definitely doing this on purpose to annoy me. They are out to get me'. 'If I don't beat them up, they will beat me up'.

The 'Hot Cross Bun'

Activity

Our emotions, sensations, thoughts and behaviours are all connected. We can get 'stuck' in a loop that keeps a problem going. Consider your main challenge that you wanted to focus on (e.g. hitting others, avoiding things, getting excluded…). What emotions, sensations, thoughts and behaviours are part of this loop?

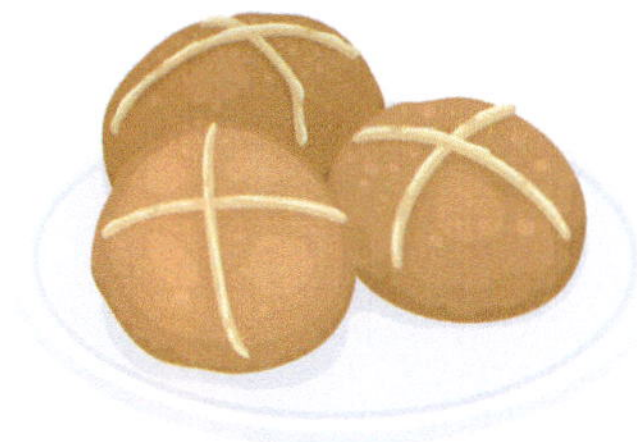

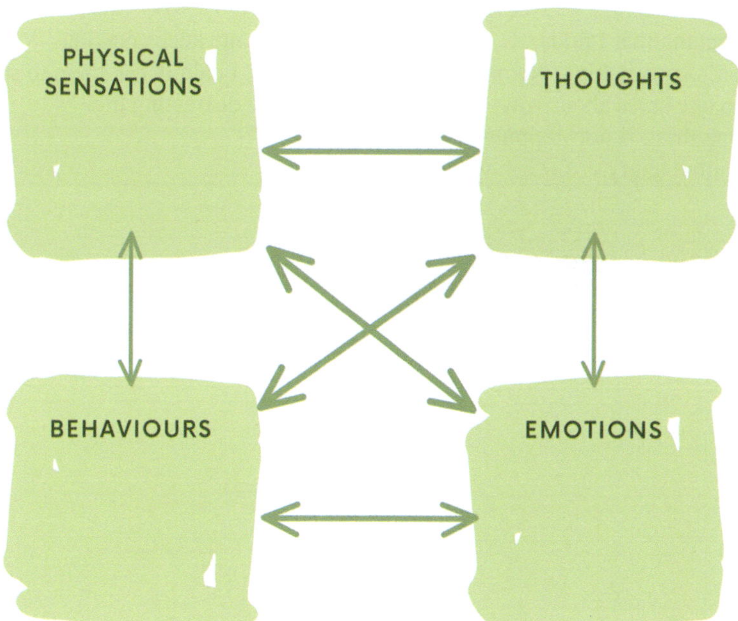

Figure 19.5

HOT thoughts and behaviours make the **emotion more intense** and keep us stuck in a loop. 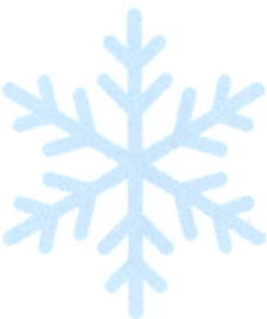 *Figure 14.2*	**COOL thoughts and behaviours** help the **emotion** be **less intense** and help us break the loop.  *Figure 14.3*
Thought 1: Everything in my life is awful. Thought 2: What is the point in trying?	Thought: I'm not sure I can handle this situation by myself, but I am going to try my best. I can also ask for help from...
1. I get annoyed at someone online so I keep talking to them and arguing. They argue back and it is getting me more and more angry. 2. Something is happening that I find annoying but I don't say anything. No one is asking me so no one cares about how I feel. The annoying thing is not stopping so I get more and more angry.	I get annoyed at someone online. They are not listening to me so I just block them and play with someone else. The person next to me keeps making annoying noises. I calmly ask them to stop because they are distracting me.

Thought Diary

Thought diaries can help us **look back** on **what happened** in our day and **challenge** how we **responded** in **difficult situations.**
They are a helpful tool to help us **understand** how our **thoughts, feelings** and **behaviours** all link together.
Reviewing situations like this can help us spot any **patterns** in how we **respond** to **difficult things**, but also **celebrate** if we **act positively** in a difficult situation.

Activity

- **Complete** the **thought diary** throughout the week. There are some **options** on **when** to **use the diary**:
    - At the **end** of the **day**: This may be **useful if** you still **struggle to stop and think** when you are in a difficult situation, or if you **struggle to find time** in the day to stop and think. At the end of the day you can **choose one important moment** or difficult situation and **think about it** when writing the diary.
    - When you are **in** a **difficult situation**: This may be **useful** to **practice stopping and thinking** before acting. If you **realise** you are **in** a **difficult situation** (e.g. angry at someone, anxious about something…) try to **take a break** from the situation, **go** to a **quiet place,** and **fill in** this **thought diary**. This may help you **decide what to do**, so you can **act** in a way that is **kinder** and more **helpful** for your goals.
- Use the columns to fill in **what happened**, your **thoughts, emotions, physical feelings** and **behaviours.**
- Use the **last column** to **reflect** on if you could have **responded differently.**

What happened? - Describe the situation -**Where** were you? - **Who** were you with?	**Thoughts** -**Unhelpful** thoughts -**Helpful** thoughts	**Emotions** -What were they? - Intensity? **0-10**	**Physical Feelings** - (e.g. stomach ache/ heart beating quickly)	**Behaviour** -What did **you do?**	Could I have **thought** or **done** something **differently?** - Any **thinking errors?** - What will I **change** for **next time?** - What **helped** that I can use again?

Communicating with Others

Communication helps us understand the world and be understood by others, it can help us express what we need and negotiate ways of getting it. However, there are many things that can affect our communication. What someone says, may not be the same as what they mean. The same can happen to us. We might try to say something, but if it is not well communicated, it may not be understood well by others.

What can affect our communication...?

- Our history/experiences
- Our social influences, for example, family, friends
- Communication channel
- Message
- Non-verbal communication, for example, gestures, facial expressions
- Mood/emotion
- Thinking errors
- Many more…

Being aware of these factors can help us plan for better communication.

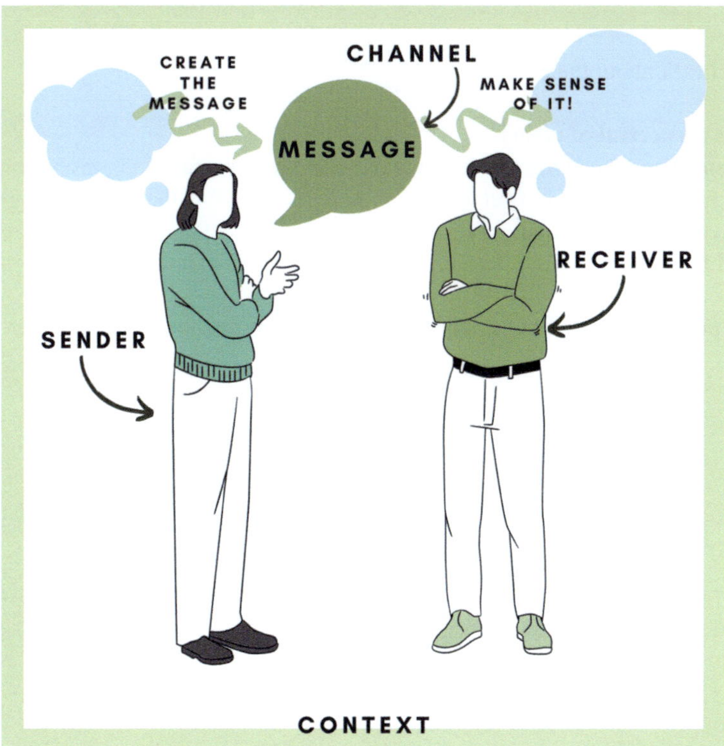

Figure 19.6

Being aware of our communication style is also important, so we can communicate in a respectful and effective way.

Being **assertive** is very important. When we are assertive we **value our** own **needs**, and **also** the **needs of others**. This allows us to **say what we need** whilst being **respectful** and **kind** to others.

What does **my assertive self** look like?

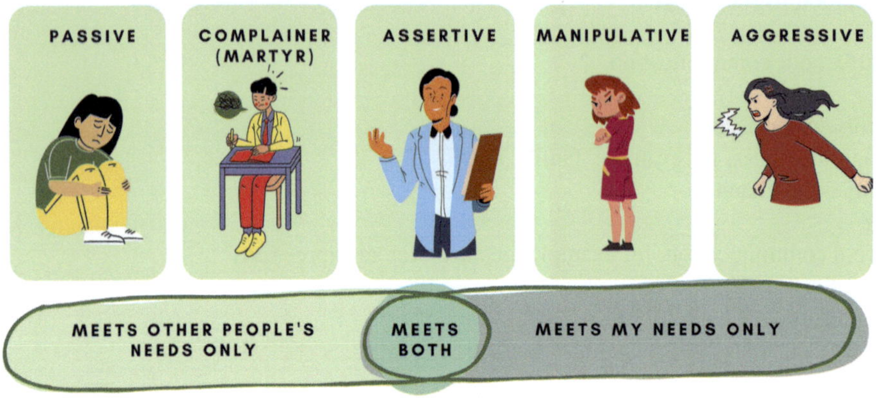

Figure 19.7

- I **value my needs** and I **talk** about them.
- I am **open** and **honest**.
- My **communication** is **respectful** of others.
- I am **calm** and **confident**. People can see this in the way I stand and my facial expressions.
- I **keep a safe distance** from others, I don't get too close – people might find that intimidating!
- I keep a **calm tone of voice**, I don't shout.
- I try **to choose a good time** for the **conversation**, so that everyone is calm and has enough time to talk.
- I **listen to** what **other people** say and I **negotiate** so their needs and my needs are both met.

Planning a Conversation

1. **What** is the **situation**? Who, what, where…
2. Goal: **What** do I **want** to **achieve**? What do I want or need?
3. How do I want to achieve my goal?

   - **What** do I want to **say**?
   - **How** do I want to **say** it?
   - **When** do I want to **say** it?

4. What **challenges** might come up?

   - Getting angry or upset
   - Getting interrupted
   - The other person disagreeing…

5. **How** can I **overcome** them?

   - Strategies…
   - Help from others…

Remember Your Strengths

Write answers to these prompts.
The most **important things** that I have **learned** in **SHERBET**:

Something I have **learned** or realised in **SHERBET** that I **do not** want to **forget**:
For example, coping skills, something helpful/unhelpful I do...

Something I **did well/achieved** in SHERBET:

Remember the things you have achieved so far!
Keep working towards your goals – you can do it!
S.H.E.R.B.E.T.

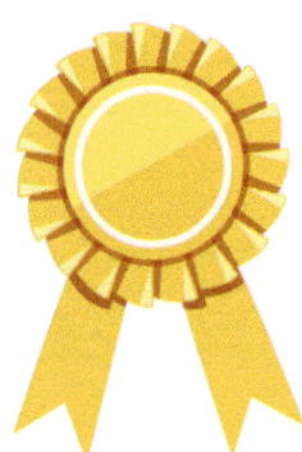

Figure 19.8

Index

For Product Safety Concerns and Information please contact our
EU representative GPSR@taylorandfrancis.com Taylor & Francis
Verlag GmbH, Kaufingerstraße 24, 80331 München, Germany